Psychotherapy

Psychotherapy

An Introduction for Psychiatry Residents and Other Mental Health Trainees

PHILLIP R. SLAVNEY, M.D.

FOREWORD BY JEROME L. KROLL, M.D.

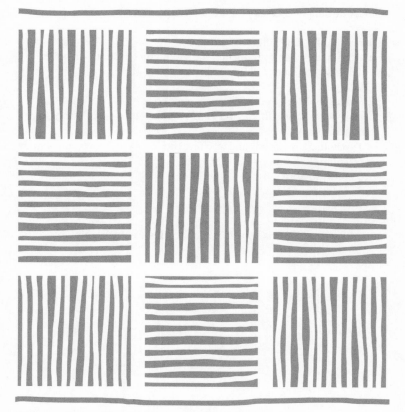

The Johns Hopkins University Press

Baltimore and London

© 2005 The Johns Hopkins University Press
All rights reserved. Published 2005
Printed in the United States of America on acid-free paper
9 8 7 6 5 4 3 2 1

The Johns Hopkins University Press
2715 North Charles Street
Baltimore, Maryland 21218-4363
www.press.jhu.edu

Library of Congress Cataloging-in-Publication Data

Slavney, Phillip R. (Phillip Richard), 1940–
    Psychotherapy : an introduction for psychiatry residents and other
mental health trainees / Phillip R. Slavney.
        p. cm.
    Includes bibliographical references and index.
    ISBN 0-8018-8095-5 (hardcover : alk. paper) — ISBN 0-8018-8096-3
(pbk. : alk. paper)
    1. Psychotherapy—Study and teaching (Residency) 2. Psychiatry—Study
and teaching (Residency) I. Title.
    RC459.S528 2005
    616.89'14'071—dc22

                                                                2004022315

A catalog record for this book is available from the British Library.

For Jacqueline

Contents

Foreword

The Accreditation Council of Graduate Medical Education (ACGME) has mandated that psychiatry residents receive training and experience and demonstrate competence in five "forms" (I would sooner say "domains") of treatment: brief therapy, cognitive-behavioral therapy, combined psychotherapy and psychopharmacology, psychodynamic therapy, and supportive therapy. Is this realistic? How can it be done in a four-year curriculum crowded with competing demands such as clinical diagnoses and the expanding body of biological knowledge and treatments that threaten to sweep aside all other considerations? Is the demand that residents (and practicing psychiatrists) master not one but five forms of psychotherapy a piece of desperate bravado in the face of twenty-first century neuroscientific hegemony, a modern imitation of King Canute's apocryphal command to the tides to cease their movement?

It might be proper for residency requirements to speak to the ideals of training and education, ranging from ethical issues and the basics of interviewing to diagnosing and the medical approach to the psychiatric patient, including all the virtues of consideration and attentiveness entailed in the Hippocratic or Maimonedean Oath. But providing experience, training, and supervision in the various forms of psychotherapy is a practical issue requiring a practical solution. The whole thrust of psychiatric practice is not conducive to a more leisurely approach in which the psychiatrist is expected to listen to the patient, make sense of the patient's troubles from that person's point of view, and help the patient develop perspective, some strategies for change, and a cause for hope. Yet somehow this must be done, not particularly because the ACGME mandates it, but because the abilities to listen with skill and to intervene with compassion are at the very core of our professional existence.

It seems to me that even if many of our future psychiatrists do not plan to or will not be in a position to do much psychotherapy in the old-fashioned formal sense, the teaching of psychotherapy constitutes the foundation of how to understand the troubles and desperation that bring patients to a psychiatrist. Some may opt for a future of computerized symptom checklists, the generation of a coded diagnosis, and the development of an algorithm for the proper medication. This capability cannot be far off, if it is not here already. But this is not what most people want when they seek a psychiatrist and it is not what most young physicians are interested in when they choose psychiatry for their life's work. I tell my medical students and residents that, ideally, at the end of a good interview or therapy session, they should have enough sense about the patient as a person to be able to write a short story about the individual for the *New Yorker* if they had the writing skills.

Phillip R. Slavney's book advances this ideal into the realm of the practical. He correctly perceives that the initial problem in teaching therapy is not to teach particular bits of technique but to provide a framework for examining the very process of therapy and to find the features common to all therapies. This primer on the basics of psychotherapy is the natural outgrowth of Paul R. McHugh and Slavney's remarkable book *The Perspectives of Psychiatry,* which analyzes the overlapping but different conditions constituting the subject matter of psychiatry: diseases, dimensions (temperament and personality), behaviors, and life stories. Each model carries its own theoretical constructs, methodology, and focus of treatment. The competent psychiatrist must apportion and integrate these approaches when providing care for the single unity that matters: the individual patient.

Interwoven throughout the fabric of this book is a central problem for beginning as well as accomplished therapists: what to do with oneself in the process of psychotherapy. Issues of boundaries, dress, office setting, and the cardinal role of not exploiting the patient for one's own benefit or satisfaction are fully and richly discussed. Slavney also addresses the details of how to do the necessary pointing out or confrontational (that awful

word) work in therapy without coming off as criticizing or attacking the patient. This is probably the rock on which much
psychotherapy is shipwrecked, but finding the proper wording,
tone, and prefatory words do not come easily. Even this skill is
interdependent on the relationship between the patient's narrative and the therapist's narrative, for the distance and discrepancy between these two most likely set up the basis for misunderstandings and problems in exchanges that are less than
empathic.

Slavney also emphasizes the importance of the relationship
and collaborative work between the resident and therapy supervisor. This crucial piece of psychotherapy training is often dealt
with in a casual manner. Residents and other trainees usually
solve the problem of a mismatch in supervisory assignment or
of an intrusive or incompetent supervisor by avoidance and
other pathways of least resistance. But if a resident averages two
psychotherapy supervisors a year, a bad experience in this major
portion of training seriously compromises learning opportunities, serves as poor role modeling, and can affect the resident's
own morale and enthusiasm for psychotherapy.

All in all, this slim book fills an important niche in the training of the twenty-first century psychiatrist. It provides a thought-
ful overview of where psychotherapy fits into the overall schema
of psychiatric training and practice, and it offers the tools for establishing therapeutic relationships with the great variety of distressed patients who seek competent and professional psychiatric care.

Jerome L. Kroll, M.D.
Professor, Department of Psychiatry
University of Minnesota Medical School

Preface and Acknowledgments

Many psychiatry residents begin their careers as psychothera-pists with a mixture of excitement and apprehension: excite-ment at the prospect of relying only on words and actions to help someone in distress; apprehension about whether they are ca-pable of doing it. In part, their doubts arise because almost noth-ing they have learned in medical school gives them confidence that they can practice psychotherapy. How much theory—and what kind—should they learn at the start? Do they have to un-dergo psychotherapy themselves to be good psychotherapists? How much personal information should they reveal to their pa-tients? I hope this book will help residents answer such ques-tions by drawing their attention to some fundamental principles of psychotherapy and to some attitudes and practices of suc-cessful psychotherapists.

Although I have written the book primarily for psychiatry res-idents, much of its content is relevant to the experience of be-ginning psychotherapists in psychology, social work, and nurs-ing. I trust that readers from disciplines other than medicine will forgive me for addressing the group of students whose ed-ucational backgrounds, clinical challenges, and ethical conflicts I understand best.

The book has grown out of my experience as a psychotherapy supervisor and psychiatry residency program director. Its focus is on individual psychotherapy with adult patients. It is not con-cerned with exploring the strengths and weaknesses of various psychotherapeutic methods, nor with all of the issues that can arise over the course of treatment. My goal is to help beginners get started, and my approach is often conversational, as if I were supervising a resident face to face. I have used quotations lib-erally, both to let the authors speak for themselves and to en-courage students of psychotherapy to read more broadly in the field.

I am grateful to Jason Brandt, Michael Clark, Paul Costa, Chandlee Dickey, Wendy Harris, Francis Mondimore, Gerald Nestadt, Jack Samuels, Martin Schneider, Jan Scott, Everett Siegel, and Jacqueline Slavney for providing information and advice; to Mark Teitelbaum for helping me define the scope of the book; and to Niccolo Della Penna and Anisa Cott for reading and commenting on the manuscript. I owe a special debt of gratitude to Jerome Kroll, Paul McHugh, and Werner Nathan for being my psychotherapy supervisors.

Psychotherapy

1. Life-Story Reasoning

Life Stories

When you ask patients why they have entered treatment, they often describe an unpleasant mood or disturbing behavior. As you ask them to elaborate, your questions and their answers generate the beginning of a story, with characters, a setting, and a sequence of events:

Psychiatrist: What's troubling you the most?
Patient: I just keep getting angry all the time.
Psychiatrist: Angry at who?
Patient: Everybody.
Psychiatrist: Everybody?
Patient: Well, mostly people at work, but I get angry at my wife, too. At work I don't say anything, but at home sometimes I shout.
Psychiatrist: Have you ever hit your wife when you've been angry?
Patient: No, but once I walked out in the middle of an argument because I was afraid I'd hit her.
Psychiatrist: When did all this start?
Patient: About six months ago, after I got a new boss. My old boss was transferred and a guy I used to work with got promoted. He just keeps the pressure on—he doesn't care how the job is done.

As you gather more information, the patient assigns motivations to the characters involved (e.g., "The boss is trying to get me out of there because I won't do things his way") and you begin to see possible themes in the story, themes linked to the patient's personality (e.g., obsessive-compulsive traits make it hard for him to change his work habits) or to events or relationships in his past (e.g., he is reacting to his new boss in the same way he reacted to his older brother). As you challenge the patient's assumptions about himself and others, as you ask his opinion about the accuracy of your interpretations, the developing story makes his distress increasingly understandable to both of you. This shared understanding of why he feels what he feels and why he does what he does becomes the basis for change.

The story that results from this process—a life story [114, pp. 253–67]—is a plausible, chronological, coherent narrative that accounts for the patient's distress. Although life stories are based on information provided by the patient, in the last analysis they are told by the psychotherapist, who not only edits what the patient reports but also suggests themes the patient has not considered.

A Most Natural Way of Reasoning

Storytelling is a very natural way of accounting for human emotions and behaviors. Cultures, religions, nations, families, and individuals all have their stories. We grow up wanting to hear stories and to tell them. In fact, as Fritz Heider and Marianne Simmel discovered [75], stories can be told about emotions and behaviors even when there are none. Heider and Simmel asked 34 college students to describe what happened in a brief film of three geometrical shapes in motion (fig. 1). Only one subject reported the events in geometrical terms:

A large solid triangle is shown entering a rectangle. It enters and comes out of this rectangle, and each time the corner and one-half of one of the sides of the rectangle form an opening. Then another, smaller triangle and a circle appear on the scene. The circle enters the rectangle while the larger triangle is within. The two move about in a circular motion and then the circle goes out of the opening and joins the smaller triangle which has been moving around outside the rectangle. Then the smaller triangle and the circle move about together and when the larger triangle comes out of the rectangle and

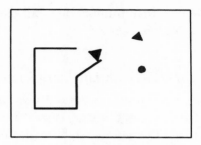

Fig. 1. Geometrical objects whose movements were described in terms of a story. *Source*: Fritz Heider and Marianne Simmel, "An Experimental Study of Apparent Behavior," *American Journal of Psychology* 57 (1944): 243–59. Copyright 1944 by the Board of Trustees of the University of Illinois. Used with permission of the University of Illinois Press.

approaches them, they move rapidly in a circle around the rectangle and disappear. [p. 246]

The other 33 subjects described the figures' movements as the actions of animate beings: in 31 cases, of people; in two cases, of birds. Nineteen subjects told a connected story about these shapes in motion. One such story began:

A man has planned to meet a girl and the girl comes along with another man. The first man tells the second to go. . . . Then the two men have a fight, and the girl starts to go into the room to get out of the way and hesitates and finally goes in. She apparently does not want to be with the first man. The first man follows her into the room after having left the second in a rather weakened condition leaning on the wall outside the room. The girl gets worried and races from one corner to the other in the far part of the room. Man number one, after being rather silent for a while, makes several approaches at her; but she gets to the corner across from the door, just as man number two is trying to open it. . . . The girl gets out of the room in a sudden dash just as man number two gets the door open. The two chase around the outside of the room together, followed by man number one. But they finally elude him and get away. [pp. 246–47]

Two Potential Problems with Life-Story Reasoning

Because life-story reasoning is so natural a way of thinking, we tend to accept it uncritically. The story carries us along as we tell it, and once its major themes are established, almost any development can be made consistent with them. For this reason, it is important to note two potential problems with the method: erroneous information and inappropriate interpretations.

Erroneous Information. If a life story is supposed to be based on an accurate recounting of actual events, then one potential problem is that the information provided by the patient is wrong. This could happen, for example, because the patient's memory for an event has faded, or because the patient's explanation of someone else's motivation is incorrect. Although in many medical settings you can increase the accuracy of information about patients by speaking to other informants, in outpatient psychotherapy you often rely on the patient alone. Not infrequently this is because the patient has troubled relationships with relatives or friends and does not want you influenced by their version of events. Still, if the patient agrees, you should seek information from other informants about the patient's personality and crucial events in his or her life. When patients are the sole informants, you should believe them, but not uncritically.

Inappropriate Interpretations. All psychotherapists have some point of view as the basis for making life-story interpretations [114, pp. 255–8]. Although as a beginning psychotherapist you may think this statement does not apply to you, it does. Your point of view to date has been derived in varying degrees from your experience of life (e.g., whether you have children), from what you learned at university and in medical school about psychological and psychiatric theories (e.g., whether you believe that unconscious conflicts produce "neurotic" illness), from your political opinions (e.g., whether you are a feminist), from your religious beliefs (e.g., whether you consider homosexuality a sin), and so on. Having a point of view is a potential problem because the goal of making interpretations in psychotherapy is to persuade patients to change how they think and act. If your point of view leads you to make interpretations that are unacceptable to the patient, the patient may leave treatment; if your point of view leads you to make inaccurate interpretations, the patient may not improve.

Same Patient, Different Stories

Psychotherapists with different points of view can interpret the same information in different ways and therefore produce different life stories for the same patient. An example of this phenomenon is the case of Anna O., which Josef Breuer [22], Sigmund Freud [48], and Marc Hollender [84] each interpreted from a different point of view. Indeed, a single psychotherapist whose point of view changes over time can tell two different stories about the same patient, as Heinz Kohut did in "The Two Analyses of Mr. Z" [98]. When Kohut treated the patient for the first time, he interpreted Mr. Z.'s childhood masturbation in terms of classical psychoanalysis; when he treated the patient for the second time, Kohut was developing his theory of self-psychology. This new point of view led him to decide that the patient's masturbation "was not drive-motivated; was not the vigorous action of the pleasure-seeking firm self of a healthy child. It was [instead] his attempt, through stimulation of the most sensitive zones of his body, to obtain temporarily the reassurance of being alive, of existing" [p. 17].

You can tell different stories for the same patient because you have to connect events in a meaningful way to have a story at all. What supplies the meaning is your point of view, and the meaningful connections you make are the glue that holds the story together. As you will see in the next section, the characteristics of meaningful connections give life-story reasoning both its capacity to find a variety of themes in an individual case and its propensity to spawn competing "schools" of psychotherapy with differing points of view.

Meaningful Connections

Karl Jaspers, the foremost student of psychiatric methodology, distinguished between meaningful connections, which are characteristic of reasoning in the humanities and social sciences, and causal connections, which are characteristic of reasoning in the natural sciences [91, 1:302–3].

Causal connections answer the *how* question, as in, "How did this patient get Huntington's disease?" Causal connections are established by a process of observation, quantification, correlation, and experimentation, and they produce answers such as: "Someone gets Huntington's disease by inheriting a mutant gene on the short arm of chromosome 4 which contains an expanded sequence of CAG trinucleotides." In this type of reasoning, patients are regarded as organisms to which things happen.

Meaningful connections answer the *why* question, as in, "Why does this patient with Huntington's disease want to have children even though she knows they will be at 50 percent risk to inherit the disorder?" Although observation, quantification, correlation, and experimentation can help establish such connections when populations are being studied, communication and empathy are needed when individuals are being treated. The answers produced by meaningful connections to the *why* question posed above might include: "Because she thinks she will be a burden to her husband in the future and wants there to be someone to help him"; "Because she has always wanted to be a mother and is thinking more in terms of her own life than that of her child." In this type of reasoning, patients are regarded as selves with emotions, aspirations, and intentions.

Characteristics of Meaningful Connections

Jaspers proposed six characteristics of meaningful connections [91, 1:356–59]. I will briefly review each of them, as well as a seventh suggested by Paul McHugh.

Meaningful Connections Are Interpretations, Even When Based on Observation. Meaningful connections reflect the significance of events to observers. For example, a father and mother can see different meanings in the announcement by their daughter that she wants to move out of the family home when she starts attending a local college: to one parent, the daughter's decision is to be encouraged as an age-appropriate development; to the other, it is to be resisted because she is too inexperienced for independent living.

In the clinical setting, it is not uncommon for members of the treatment team to draw different conclusions from the same observation on morning rounds: to you, an inpatient's request for a pass to visit relatives so that he can mend some fences is a sign that he wants to address the interpersonal difficulties you have been discussing with him in individual psychotherapy; to another staff member, his request is a manipulative excuse to avoid group psychotherapy, where another patient has been confronting him about his exaggerated sense of importance.

Meaningful Connections Follow the "Hermeneutic Round." Jaspers proposed that the interpretations we make are determined to some extent by premises we already hold; once those interpretations are made, the premises are strengthened and elaborated. This constitutes the "hermeneutic round." We usually think of the term *hermeneutics* in the context of scriptural exegesis, but it can be used to refer to the interpretation of any text, including a life story.

All interpretations begin with a premise or point of view. A Christian reading the Bible, for example, starts with the belief that Jesus was the Messiah, so prophecies about the Messiah in the book of Isaiah are thought, quite naturally, to refer to Jesus. The Christian reader's ability to make that interpretation strengthens his or her belief that Jesus was the Christ. A Jew reading Isaiah starts with a different premise and so interprets prophecies about the Messiah as unfulfilled—so far.

When psychotherapists propose meaningful connections in a life story, those connections also follow the hermeneutic round. Thus, for example, if we start with the premise that compulsions represent a need for control, the discovery of compul-

sions in a patient's history prompts us to interpret other phenomena (e.g., the patient's refusal to delegate responsibility) as
manifestations of that same need.

Opposite Connections Are Equally Meaningful. When meaningful connections are presented in the abstract, opposite connections are equally meaningful. It is just as plausible to say, for
example, that people tell jokes about their own ethnic group because they are secretly ashamed of their identity as it is to say
that they tell such jokes because they have completely accepted
their culture, foibles and all.

This characteristic of meaningful connections is illustrated by
the contrasting theories of Wilhelm Reich and Judd Marmor on
the genesis of the "hysterical" personality [166, p. 183]. Reich
proposed that "the hysterical character is determined by a fixa-
tion in the genital stage of childhood development, with its
incestuous attachment" and that if oral fixations play a role,
"they are embodiments of genitality or at least allied with it" [143,
p. 206]. Although Marmor did not deny "the tremendous and
unquestionable part which oedipal fixations play in the hys-
teric," he believed that "a review of the clinical material in most
cases will reveal that the fixations in the oedipal phase of development are *themselves the outgrowths of preoedipal fixations, chiefly
of an oral nature*" [123, p. 662].

In the past, psychotherapists often became partisans (and
sometimes casualties) in the theoretical struggles generated by
this and other characteristics of meaningful connections. With
increased understanding of what successful psychotherapists
have in common, however, and with increased emphasis on
practical, rather than theoretical, issues in psychotherapy, this
danger has diminished. Beginning psychotherapists would do
well to remember that, given the nature of meaningful connections, an argument in the abstract can be made for almost any
point of view, including one opposite to that which you hold. The
corrective to this in an individual case is to ground your interpretations, so far as possible, in an accurate history and dispassionate observation.

Meaningful Connections Are Incomplete. Our knowledge of

other people is fragmentary. Many of their thoughts, moods, and behaviors are determined by things of which we are unaware. We sometimes have evidence of this phenomenon in psychotherapy when we make a meaningful connection between past events and current emotions and the patient corrects us by providing additional history that casts those emotions in a new light. Another reason that meaningful connections are incomplete is that some of them start with phenomena (e.g., the occurrence of puberty, the onset of hallucinations) that cannot be understood empathically but must be explained scientifically. Finally, meaningful connections are incomplete because we cannot know the future. Something unexpected can happen in a patient's life (e.g., he or she falls in love) and that event writes a new chapter, with new themes, in the story.

Meaningful Connections Are Unlimited in Number. Breuer, Freud, and Hollender each proposed a different interpretation for the case of Anna O. Given that meaningful connections are unlimited in number, it should not be surprising that more could be found, as Max Rosenbaum and Melvin Muroff discovered in their book *Anna O.: Fourteen Contemporary Reinterpretations* [146]. This characteristic of meaningful connections might lead you to think that, for a particular patient, the choice of one interpretation rather than another is trivial. Not so, wrote Jaspers: "As soon as we believe we can make some definite interpretation, another presents itself. . . . It lies in the very essence of meaningfulness. . . . On the other hand, as empirically accessible material grows, understanding becomes more decisive. Multiplicity does not necessarily imply haphazard uncertainty but can mean a flexible movement within the range of possibility that leads to an increasing certainty of vision" [91, 1:358–59].

A corollary of this characteristic of meaningful connections is that you should become familiar with a variety of theoretical approaches to psychotherapeutic interpretation. One approach (e.g., an Adlerian emphasis on striving to overcome feelings of inferiority) might be appropriate for Patient A, while another approach (e.g., a Sullivanian focus on anxiety in interpersonal relations) seems more apt for Patient B. Your ability to think in terms of various theories should increase with experience in psychotherapy, with supervision by teachers who have differing perspectives, and with your own reading in the field. Eventually, you should be able to employ several approaches to interpretation, depending on the particulars of the case, rather than always taking the same approach, no matter what.

Meaningful Connections Both Illuminate and Expose. The final characteristic Jaspers proposed for meaningful connections contrasts a sympathetic appreciation of human beings and their predicaments ("illumination") with a tendency to see through behavior and reduce it to nothing but the expression of some hidden—and often base—motivation ("exposure"). An example of such contrasting use of meaningful connections is found in the views of Johann Wolfgang von Goethe and Sigmund Freud on why Hamlet hesitates to kill Claudius and thereby avenge his father's murder.

For Goethe, Hamlet is a sensitive young man, dismayed by the enormity of what he must do:

> And when the ghost has vanished, what do we see standing before us? A young hero thirsting for revenge? A prince by birth, happy to be charged with unseating the usurper of his throne? Not at all! Amazement and sadness descend on this lonely spirit; he becomes bitter at the smiling villains, swears not to forget his departed father, and ends with a heavy sigh: "The time is out of joint; O cursed spite! That ever I was born to set it right!"
>
> In these words, so I believe, lies the key to Hamlet's whole behavior; and it is clear to me what Shakespeare set out to portray: a heavy deed placed on a soul which is not adequate to cope with it. And it is in this sense that I find the whole play constructed. . . .
>
> A fine, pure, noble and highly moral person, but devoid of that emotional strength that characterizes a hero, goes to pieces beneath a burden that it can neither support nor cast off. Every obligation is sacred to him, but this one is too heavy. The impossible is demanded of him—not the impossible in

any absolute sense, but what is impossible for him. How he twists and turns, trembles, advances and retreats, always being reminded, always reminding himself, and finally almost losing sight of his goal, yet without ever regaining happiness! [62, p. 146]

For Freud, the explanation of Hamlet's hesitation is quite different: the Oedipus complex—something that explains not only Hamlet's behavior but Shakespeare's as well:

The play is built up on Hamlet's hesitations over fulfilling the task of revenge that is assigned to him; but the text offers no reasons or motives for these hesitations and an immense variety of attempts at interpreting them have failed to produce a result. According to the view which was originated by Goethe and is still the prevailing one to-day, Hamlet represents the type of man whose power of direct action is paralysed by an excessive development of his intellect. (He is "sicklied o'er with the pale cast of thought.") . . . The plot of the drama shows us, however, that Hamlet is far from being represented as a person incapable of taking any action. We see him doing so on two occasions: first in a sudden outburst of temper, when he runs his sword through the eavesdropper behind the arras. . . . What is it, then, that inhibits him in fulfilling the task set him by his father's ghost? The answer, once again, is that it is the peculiar nature of the task. Hamlet is able to do anything—except take vengeance on the man who did away with his father and took that father's place with his mother, the man who shows him the repressed wishes of his own childhood realized. Thus the loathing which should drive him on to revenge is replaced in him by self-reproaches, by scruples of conscience, which remind him that he himself is literally no better than the sinner whom he is to punish. Here I have translated into conscious terms what was bound to remain unconscious in Hamlet's mind. . . . It can of course only be the poet's own mind which confronts us in Hamlet. . . . [which] was written immediately after the death of Shakespeare's father (in 1601), that is, under the impact of his bereavement and, as we may well assume, while his childhood feelings about his father had been freshly revived. [46, pp. 264–65]

Jaspers condemned the thoughtless use of meaningful connections in a reductive, exposing way. One should not, of course, gloss over traits (e.g., antisocial) or behaviors (e.g., lying) that cause trouble for the patient and others, but neither should one reduce the complexity of the patient's plight to the manifestation of some repressed phenomenon (e.g., castration anxiety).

Meaningful Connections in the Abstract Are Maxims, Not Laws. To the six characteristics of meaningful connections that Jaspers proposed, Paul McHugh has added a seventh [167]. This property can be seen when meaningful connections are presented in the abstract, as part of a theory about psychiatric illness. In this form, meaningful connections that were seen to occur in the lives of a few patients are presented as if they occur in the lives of many. Thus, for example, Fritz Perls wrote:

All neurotic disturbances arise from the individual's inability to find and maintain the proper balance between himself and the rest of the world, and all of them have in common the fact that in neurosis the social and environmental boundary is felt as extending too far over into the individual. The neurotic is the man on whom society impinges too heavily. His *neurosis* is a defensive maneuver to protect himself against the threat of being crowded out by an overwhelming world. [135, p. 31]

An abstract meaningful connection such as "The neurotic is the man on whom society impinges too heavily" is not a law of nature but rather a maxim or proverb. Like the saying "Absence makes the heart grow fonder," it is true in certain instances, but by no means all. Abstract meaningful connections are useful in providing concise statements of potential themes in life stories, but they must not be given more weight than that. The predicaments that bring patients to psychotherapy are too complex to be summed up in a sentence.

Narrative Truth

In its first telling, a life story is incomplete—not so much because patients cannot remember everything but because they cannot explain everything. Patients ask for help not in establishing the exact sequence of events in the past but in understanding why they are thinking, feeling, or acting as they are in the present. The answers you give to these *why* questions are framed in terms of meaningful connections between the patient's personality and his or her background and current situation. Such connections fill gaps in the story and enable it to provide a coherent understanding of the problem.

The nature of meaning is such that several possible answers can be found for every *why* question. The best of these answers can be so convincing that you and the patient accept it as true and incorporate it into the story, even though its factual basis is difficult or impossible to establish. Thus, for example, although you attribute the patient's lack of confidence to his mother's sarcastic criticism of him when he was a child, you have no way of knowing for certain that this is the whole—or even the major— explanation for the problem. The patient's parents are dead, he has no siblings, and there are no documents from the period against which his memory can be checked. Despite your inability to prove that the connection is true in a historical sense, if it seems "right" to you and the patient it becomes true in the context of the story. This type of truth is called "narrative truth" by Donald Spence:

> Narrative truth can be defined as the criterion we use to decide when a certain experience has been captured to our satisfaction; it depends on continuity and closure and the extent to which the fit of the pieces takes on an aesthetic finality. Narrative truth is what we have in mind when we say that such

and such is a good story, that a given explanation carries con-
viction. . . . Once a given construction has acquired narrative
truth, it becomes just as real as any other kind of truth. [169,
p. 31]

Could a life story be historically false in some important way
and still be clinically useful? Up to a point, I suppose, just as the
Ptolemaic system of astronomy was scientifically false but still
useful in navigation. Still, both a false life story and a false as-
tronomical system will eventually be found wanting.

When the Ptolemaic astronomers' theory failed to account for
a growing body of observations, they did not abandon their belief that the earth was the center of the universe and that celes-
tial objects moved in perfect circles around it [105, pp. 64–72].
Instead, they resorted to computational gymnastics (e.g., drawing small circles on the circumference of large circles) to preserve the principle of circular orbits and make their observations
"come out right."

If the life story you tell is rejected by the patient or is not helping to produce symptomatic improvement, one of the things you
should question is the story itself. Psychotherapists who refuse
to do this sometimes go through conceptual gymnastics rather
than revise the story. You may, for example, believe that a patient
works long hours at her job in order to overcome feelings of inferiority. If the patient denies it and says that she works hard because her job is challenging and enjoyable, you may be tempted
to say that she is using the defense mechanism of rationaliza-
tion. In this way, no matter what the patient says or does, the
theme of overcoming inferiority can be preserved. I am not saying here that patients never rationalize; I am saying that you
must think critically about the story you tell and be prepared to
reconsider its themes as you learn more about the patient.

This tentative attitude about an evolving life story is important because the use of narrative truth in psychotherapy is un-
avoidable. As a psychotherapist, you are neither a scientist nor
a philosopher, but someone treating real patients in real time.
You must do your best to help those patients understand why

they are thinking, feeling, or acting as they are. In many cases, narrative truth is the best you can do because there is no way to establish historical truth independent of the patient's memory. If you have been an insightful and critical storyteller, what you propose as narrative truth may actually be historical truth, especially if the patient finds it illuminating and "right."

Evaluating Life Stories

Life stories depend on meaningful connections and narrative truth, yet meaningful connections are plastic and narrative truth is not necessarily historical truth. Under the circumstances, how can you evaluate the life stories you tell? The most obvious test is whether the patient confirms the story and uses it as a basis for change. A story that helps produce the desired result is rarely challenged.

Yet what if the story is rejected by the patient or does not contribute to the patient's improvement? Even a good story, if poorly told or overly threatening, can suffer these fates. More often, perhaps, a story fails because it is inherently flawed and leads the psychotherapist and patient astray. In order to minimize this risk, you should think critically about the story as you develop it. One set of standards for such an evaluation was suggested by Michael Sherwood [162, pp. 20–22, 244–57]. Although Sherwood was writing about psychoanalytic narratives, the three criteria he proposed are applicable to any psychotherapeutic life story.

First, the story should be *appropriate* to a particular person and situation. Even though two patients may be anxious about losing their jobs, one is a self-deprecating young laborer about to be married and the other is a narcissistic professional facing retirement from a long and successful career. These patients have a common theme in their stories but very different backgrounds and personalities. These differences will be reflected, for example, in what the job loss means to each of them and in what strengths each can muster to deal with it. The more appropriate the story is to its context, the more it is derived from an understanding of the patient's culture, upbringing, character, aspirations, and the like, the more acceptable and useful it will be.

The second criterion Sherwood proposed for evaluating life stories is *adequacy*. By this he meant that the story should be self-consistent, coherent, and comprehensive. A story gains these properties as you use meaningful connections and narrative truth to resolve inconsistencies, link themes, and fill gaps. The story that results has a beginning (how the patient came to develop the troubles he or she now has); a middle (why the patient's attempts to deal with those troubles have failed); and an end (how the patient's understanding of what has gone before now enables him or her to make wiser choices, have more realistic goals, and so on).

The last of Sherwood's criteria is *accuracy*. One way to judge this is whether the story is consistent with your observations of the patient. If, for example, a patient lacks assertiveness in psychotherapy, he or she might be expected to show the same trait in other situations. If that were true, the trait might be used to explain certain problems and could be a prominent theme in the story. If the patient denies being unassertive, the discrepancy between what you observe and what the patient reports must be resolved.

Sherwood also proposed that stories are accurate to the extent that they are consistent with truths about individuals who are similar to the patient and consistent with what he called "general truths about human behavior" [p. 255]. A truth about similar individuals might be that a patient is easily bored because he or she is an extravert, and extraverts quickly tire of routine. A "general truth about human behavior" might be that grief follows the loss of a close relationship.

Checking a story's consistency with your observations of the patient is relatively easy, not only because you see the patient again and again but also because, in some instances, other informants can validate or refute those observations. Checking a story's consistency with truths about similar individuals can present a greater problem, depending on how you know what those other individuals are like. If your patient scores as an extravert on the Revised NEO Personality Inventory [30], for example, you can be reasonably confident that he or she is like other extraverts in certain regards [112], perhaps including being easily bored [81]. When the similar individual is represented by a single patient (another of yours, a supervisor's, or one described in the literature), however, exercise caution before you draw a close parallel. Even if your patient, like Anna O., is a young woman with medically unexplained complaints who has recently lost her father, whose "truth" about Anna O. would you use as a model for your case: that of Breuer, Freud, Hollender, or another interpreter altogether? Patients *are* similar in certain ways, and your knowledge of such similarities will make you a more efficient and effective psychotherapist, but you should remember that even though patients are alike in some characteristics, they are quite different in others, and that their differences may be more important than their similarities.

Checking a story's consistency with a "general truth about human behavior" can be very straightforward if the "general truth" is something like "Grief follows the loss of a close relationship." Such a statement is not only a matter of everyday observation; it is also a phenomenon that has been studied empirically [97; 133]. Sometimes, however, a statement such as the following is presented as a "general truth":

> Psychoanalysts have defined a widespread, if not universal, fantasy in which, unconsciously, penis and breast are equated; and correlatively, semen and milk. These equations are especially salient in the analyses of those people who have centered their sexual interest in fellatio fantasies and practices, no matter whether they have done so in an overexcited, repulsed, or paralyzed fashion. Much gagging and vomiting of psychological origin can be attributed in part to a person's engaging in these fantasies conflictually and unconsciously. [156, p. 90]

Even if it could be shown that a certain number of patients in psychoanalysis equate the penis and the breast, no data are presented or cited to support the claim that such a fantasy is "widespread, if not universal."

As a beginner in psychotherapy, you may be so impressed by the confidence and rhetorical skill with which such ideas are presented that you uncritically include them in a life story—with unfortunate results. If you tell a patient with "psychogenic" vomiting that the complaint ipso facto represents a reaction to an unconscious fantasy about fellatio, and the patient rejects the interpretation or is insulted by it, you may be more likely to think that the patient is "denying" or "resisting" than to wonder what evidence you have to back up your opinion save that the patient is vomiting, that there is no apparent physiological explanation for it, and that you have read or heard an unsubstantiated claim about how human beings behave. If a "general truth about human behavior" is to be used as a criterion for judging the accuracy of a life story, that "general truth" should be very well supported.

2. Personality: The Patient's and Yours

Patients seek psychotherapy because they are thinking, feeling, or acting in ways that are distressing or maladaptive. At the start of the process, they usually relate their problem to a situation they are in (e.g., a deteriorating relationship, impending academic or occupational failure) and want your help changing that situation. As you take the history, however, you often discover that the patient has had difficulty with similar situations in the past, and you begin to see a pattern of troubles arising from the type of individual the patient is (e.g., dependent, antisocial). Although patients are very aware of their symptoms and their circumstances, they are sometimes much less aware of how their personalities have contributed to their problems. Part of what you do for patients, then, is to help them appreciate their vulnerabilities and strengths so that they can avoid trouble in the future and deal more effectively with it should it occur.

Although this is one important reason for you to understand the patient's personality, there is another equally important one. The patient's personality—and your personality—shape the psychotherapeutic relationship, and it is the relationship that determines the success of treatment. (This topic is further discussed in chapter 3.) If you are to maximize your effectiveness as a psychotherapist, then, you must understand not only how the patient's personality has contributed to his or her troubles, but also how it is contributing to his or her participation in treatment. You should be able to adapt your psychotherapeutic approach to the patient's personality, just as you should be able to adapt the medications you prescribe to the patient's symptoms. Before I suggest which adaptations are most appropriate for which traits, I will briefly discuss personality and its assessment.

The Concept of Traits

Personality is described in terms of cognitive, temperamental, and behavioral traits. Such traits are relatively stable character- istics or dispositions [172], so that someone who is intelligent or cheerful or courageous in one situation tends to be that way in others. Not everyone, however, is equally intelligent, cheerful, or courageous, for people differ in the degree to which they have various characteristics. Traits, then, are dimensions of variation along which individuals can be compared to one another. Just as there are gradations of height (a physical trait), there are grada- tions of intelligence (a psychological trait).

The Assessment of Traits

Although differences in height are immediately evident when we look at a group of people, differences in intelligence are not. Unlike physical traits, cognitive, temperamental, and behavioral traits need situations to reveal them. In everyday life, we can es- timate intelligence by how quickly someone grasps an abstract point; cheerfulness by how rapidly someone recovers from dis- appointment; and courage by how directly someone confronts danger. In psychotherapy, our observations of the patient are limited to the treatment setting itself. Although such observa- tions are very useful, they take time to accumulate, and we need to get a sense of the patient's personality from the outset.

Taking a Trait Inventory

The most natural way to do an initial assessment of the patient's personality is to include a trait inventory as part of the history. The goal of the assessment is to learn what the patient was like before the illness began. A good time to ask about the premor- bid personality is just after you have taken the psychiatric his- tory: "I think I've got a pretty good picture of what's troubling you now, but I also want to know what you were like before all this started—what you're like at your baseline. If you were going to describe your personality to someone else, what would you say?" By beginning in this way, you allow patients to tell you which traits they regard as their most important characteristics. When patients are at a loss to describe themselves, you could introduce the trait inventory by saying, "I think I've got a pretty good picture of what's troubling you now, but I also want to know what you were like before all this started—what you're like at your baseline. For example, would you say you're a confident person or a self-doubting one?"

The questions you ask about traits can be phrased in terms of a single characteristic (e.g., "How optimistic a person would you say you are?") or in terms of a pair of contrasting attributes (e.g., "Would you say you're more of an optimist or a pessimist?"). However you phrase the questions, you should ask about characteristics that are important in relationships or at work or school, for these are the situations in which trait-related troubles usually arise. I think the following traits are representative of those characteristics:

optimistic / pessimistic
suspicious / trusting
even-tempered / moody
worrier / carefree
controlled / demonstrative
dependent / independent
cautious / impulsive
stingy / generous
leader / follower
solitary / sociable
patient / impatient
strict / easy-going
confident / self-doubting
unreliable / reliable
easily hurt / thick-skinned
neat / messy
self-conscious / unconcerned about what others think

This list will not produce anything like a detailed self-portrait of the patient, but it will generate an initial sketch. Depending on the particulars of the case, you will want to ask about other characteristics (e.g., ambitiousness in someone whose business is failing, jealousy in someone who cannot sustain romantic relationships). As for traits that are important but may be initially awkward to ask about (e.g., honesty), you will have to rely on your own observations and, if possible, on descriptions of the patient from other informants.

One question that immediately arises about a patient's self-description is its validity. Perhaps by now you have heard an antisocial patient with a history of cruelty say that one of his outstanding characteristics is his kindness to others. It is in the matter of validity that descriptions of patients from other informants are potentially most valuable. Eventually, of course, you will be able to use your own experience with patients to judge, for some traits at least, how valid their self-descriptions are.

Using Personality Tests

Another way to obtain an initial assessment of the patient's personality is through personality tests—either questionnaires that patients complete or standardized interviews that you conduct. It is important to note at the outset that neither type of test yields information that is fundamentally different from what you would obtain with a trait inventory such as the one described above. A trait inventory, a paper-and-pencil self-report questionnaire, and a standardized interview all do the same thing: ask patients to describe themselves. Widely used personality tests can be useful because they allow you to compare the responses of your patient to those of many other individuals, but they are not like x-rays or metabolic panels—they do not reveal things about the patient you cannot otherwise see.

There are a considerable number of both self-report questionnaires and standardized interviews, but a comparative review of their strengths and weaknesses (not to mention their reliability and validity) is beyond the scope of this book. One general comment, however, is that some instruments produce scores on personality traits (e.g., neuroticism, self-discipline) as such, while others produce scores on personality categories (e.g., borderline, schizoid). To some extent this difference is that between tests developed by psychologists, who tend to favor dimensional reasoning, and tests developed by psychiatrists, who tend to favor categorical reasoning. A discussion of the differences between thinking about personality in terms of traits or dimensions and thinking about it in terms of categories or types is also beyond my purpose here, but the topic is important for psychiatrists to consider at some time in their careers [42; 114, pp. 126–37; 183].

The NEO PI-R: An Example of a Self-Report Questionnaire. Many psychologists believe that five basic trait domains—neuroticism, extraversion, openness, agreeableness, and conscientiousness—best represent the structure of personality [112]. The Revised NEO Personality Inventory (NEO PI-R) is designed to assess these domains and the specific traits ("facets") that constitute them [30]. The domain *extraversion,* for example, contains the following facets: warmth, gregariousness, assertiveness, activity, excitement-seeking, and positive emotions. The NEO PI-R consists of 240 items (e.g., "I'm pretty stable emotionally") which patients rate on a five-point scale from "strongly disagree" to "strongly agree." There is an identical form (save for the pronoun used) which can be filled out by someone who knows the patient well [113]. The NEO PI-R takes about 45 minutes to complete.

The relationship between trait scores on the NEO PI-R and personality disorder categories in the *Diagnostic and Statistical Manual of Mental Disorders* (DSM) [5] is a matter of ongoing assessment. A major point at issue is whether the five domains noted above can usefully distinguish one personality disorder category from another [109; 128; 188].

The SIDP-IV: An Example of a Standardized Interview. The Structured Interview for DSM-IV Personality (SIDP-IV) [138], contains 78 items covering the DSM-IV personality disorder categories. Most items are traits that the interviewer assesses by asking the patient one or more questions. The schizoid trait *takes pleasure in few, if any activities,* for example, is initially evaluated by the question "What kind of things do you enjoy?" If the patient lists only one or two activities, the interviewer asks, "If [those things] were not available, are there other things you would enjoy doing?" On the basis of such questions the item is scored on a four-point scale from 0 ("not present, or limited to rare, isolated examples") to 3 ("strongly present . . . associated with subjective distress or some impairment in social or occupational functioning, or intimate relationships"). A few items (e.g., the schizotypal trait *behavior or appearance that is odd, eccentric, or peculiar*) are scored by observing the patient during the interview, which takes about an hour to complete.

The SIDP-IV can also be used to obtain a description of the patient's personality from another informant. In such cases, the informant's observations of the patient are used to score traits such as the schizotypal one noted above. The SIDP-IV, like the NEO PI-R, can elicit discordant assessments from patients and other informants [15; 189].

The Interaction of Traits and Situations

If traits are dimensions of variation, a patient's position along those dimensions determines that individual's strengths and vulnerabilities in particular situations. Patient A, for example, is very intelligent but quite dependent, while Patient B is the reverse. Patient A does well in advanced placement courses in college but is very upset by the loss of a relationship that Patient B would regard as rather superficial. Patient B, in contrast, is quite resilient in the face of romantic disappointment but struggles to pass a remedial course that Patient A would find a snap. What we see, then, is a rather specific interaction between traits and situations in the production of emotional distress or maladaptive behavior.

If specificity is one aspect of the interaction between traits and situations, intensity is another [114, pp. 141–47]. The more vulnerable someone is as regards a certain trait, the less provocation is required to trigger a response. Patient A is more suspicious than Patient B and therefore needs less uncertainty before becoming anxious.

Most patients who come for psychotherapy do not do so because they are in a situation that most people would find distressing (e.g., losing all their possessions in a hurricane). Instead, they come because they are upset by the predicaments of everyday life (e.g., disciplining an unruly child, being passed over for a promotion). In some of these cases, you discover that the patient has coped well with anger or disappointment in the past and you need do little more than help the patient understand the situation better and formulate a plan for dealing with it. In other cases, however, you find a pattern of trait-situation interactions that has produced repeated difficulties for the patient and others. In these latter cases, the diagnosis of a personality disorder is usually warranted and the process of psychotherapy is more prolonged and arduous.

Although traits are relatively stable phenomena, a motivated patient can modify certain of them or at least learn to take them into account when choosing a course of action. It is difficult to study the outcome of psychotherapy for patients with personality disorders (because, for example, treatment variables are harder to control in psychotherapy than in pharmacotherapy), but such studies demonstrate that psychotherapy can be effective [12; 54; 136; 155]. Even without that confirmation, however, you will want to use psychotherapy for patients with personality disorders because you will want to help them understand why they are distressed and what they can do about it—because you care about them. In the words of Jerome Frank, "caring in this sense does not necessarily imply approval, but rather a determination to persist in trying to help, no matter how desperate patients' conditions or how outrageous their behavior. The helping alliance implies the therapist's acceptance of the sufferer, if not for what he or she is, then for what he or she can become" [44, p. 40].

How the Patient's Personality Affects the Process of Psychotherapy

Most psychiatric observations of how a patient's personality affects the process of psychotherapy have been made within the framework of personality types or categories—paranoid, narcissistic, obsessive-compulsive, and the like. In what follows I note some prominent traits in the Cluster A, B, and C personality types described by DSM-IV (table 1) and comment on how those traits shape the course of treatment. My aim is not to discuss every trait and its effect on the process of psychotherapy but to point out common trait-related problems and suggest how beginners can deal with them.

Keep in mind that traits ascribed to one personality type can also occur in another. Thus, for example, both borderline and histrionic individuals are emotionally labile. Furthermore, many patients have traits ascribed to several types. In this way, someone can be secretive (a paranoid trait), have unstable relationships (a borderline trait), and be fearful of criticism (an avoidant trait). The effect a given trait has on the process of psychotherapy will be modified to some extent by the other traits associated with it.

In what follows, I assume that patients with each personality type have sought out psychotherapy or that psychotherapy is being provided as part of the treatment of a DSM-IV Axis I condition (e.g., major depressive disorder, generalized anxiety disorder, conversion disorder). In practice, individuals with schizoid and schizotypal personalities rarely request psychotherapy, and those with paranoid and antisocial personalities are unlikely to do so.

Paranoid Personality

To a paranoid patient, the words and acts of a psychotherapist are no different from those of other individuals: phenomena to be analyzed for their potential to deceive, manipulate, or humiliate. Even though the patient has come to you for help, suspiciousness is so fundamental to his or her way of thinking that the patient must struggle to trust and confide in you. To someone as vigilant and sensitive as a paranoid person, many things are not what they seem.

David Shapiro provides an excellent illustration of the effect of paranoid thinking on the process of psychotherapy in his de-

Table 1. DSM-IV Personality Disorders

Clusters	Disorders	Some Traits Affecting Psychotherapeutic Process
A (odd/eccentric)	Paranoid	Suspiciousness Secretiveness
	Schizoid	Social detachment Emotional restriction
	Schizotypal	Self-referential thinking Odd use of language
B (dramatic/erratic)	Antisocial	Deceitfulness Aggressiveness
	Borderline	Unstable relationships Self-injurious behavior
	Histrionic	Impressionistic thinking Emotional lability
	Narcissistic	Superior self-attitude Feeling of entitlement
C (anxious/fearful)	Avoidant	Fear of being criticized Reluctance to take risks
	Dependent	Passivity Reluctance to disagree
	Obsessive- Compulsive	Preoccupation with details Doubting

Source: American Psychiatric Association. *Diagnostic and Statistical Manual of Mental Disorders, Fourth Edition.* Washington, DC: American Psychiatric Association, 1994.

scription of a patient who admitted, after some time in treatment, that his focus was not on what the psychotherapist ostensibly said but on what the psychotherapist might actually mean:

> The patient . . . like suspicious people generally, listened and watched very sharply, but he listened for something quite dif-

ferent from the normal object of interest. He listened and watched only for clues to what, according to his suppositions, the therapist might be up to. He probably noticed every unusual phrase or flicker of hesitation. But, meanwhile, the whole sense of the communication, its otherwise apparent point and substance, its face value, was correspondingly diminished for him. The suspicious person, in other words, regards a communication or a situation not to apprehend what it is, but to understand what it signifies. [161, p. 65]

Beginning psychiatry residents are very concerned about whether they are making appropriate interpretations and suggestions, but they often overlook the fact that for patients—especially paranoid ones—what is said on the way to the interpretation or suggestion may be the most important thing. In the following exchange between a psychiatrist and a paranoid patient who felt slighted by her sister, the psychiatrist wishes to interpret the patient's reaction in light of her past relationship with her sister. In order to begin the transition to that interpretation, the psychiatrist makes a bridging comment:

Psychiatrist: Most people probably wouldn't have thought your sister was ignoring you. They'd have thought she didn't see you when she first came in.
Patient: What do you mean, "most people"?
Psychiatrist: Well, I mean that most people would have thought she went to talk to your cousins first because she saw them first. The room was crowded and she might not have seen you.
Patient: How do you know what "most people" would have thought?
Psychiatrist: What I was trying to say was that there could be several reasons why your sister didn't speak to you first. I'm sorry if I wasn't clear.
Patient: Do you think I should be like "most people"? "Most people" don't have a sister like mine.
Psychiatrist: Again, I'm sorry I wasn't clear.

In this exchange, what the psychiatrist intended as an innocent transition was taken by the patient as a criticism. As a result, the psychiatrist was placed on the defensive and the conversation got further and further from the point the psychiatrist wanted to make.

There is almost no way to avoid being misunderstood by a paranoid patient, but you can reduce the potential for misunderstanding by not making offhand remarks or (what you take to be) witticisms. It is also helpful to preface certain comments with something like "What I'm going to say next is an observation, not a criticism." This encourages the patient to take the observation at face value. Similarly, before offering an interpretation you might say, "I'd like to propose one way of explaining why you might have felt like that. I don't mean it's the only way, but I'd like to know if it seems right to you." Comments such as this underline your respect for the patient and keep your options open. When you misspeak or are misunderstood, a prompt apology or clarification helps get the conversation back on track.

Because paranoid patients sometimes ask to see their medical records, it is important that you write your psychotherapy notes in such a way as to minimize the possibility of misunderstanding. You should also inform the patient when there has been a request for information (e.g., from an insurance company) and ask the patient if he or she wants to read your response before you send it [141].

Another characteristic of paranoid patients that affects the process of psychotherapy is their secretiveness. Their reluctance to confide in others means that they have difficulty fulfilling a fundamental responsibility of patients in psychotherapy—to disclose all information relevant to the problem for which they are seeking help. As they respond to your questions, paranoid patients can withhold information or lie.

Many patients in psychotherapy initially withhold some information, perhaps out of embarrassment. As the psychotherapeutic relationship develops, however, most of them are forthcoming because they come to trust you. Paranoid patients find it hard to trust anyone—even physicians—and may remain suspicious of your motives for a long time. When paranoid patients refuse to discuss a certain topic, you should explain in a matter-of-fact way the reason for your interest and then move on, with a plan to revisit the topic at a later time. Admonishing paranoid patients for withholding information can be counterproductive.

Lying is a difficult matter to deal with in any event, even when the patient does not have paranoid traits. At first, it may be difficult to tell when you are being lied to. As you get to know the patient better, however, false information is easier to discern because it is inconsistent with what you already know about the individual. In perilous situations (e.g., when the life of the patient or another person is at risk), you must confront the patient with your doubts and then, depending on the response, decide what to do as best you can. (In these cases, when time and circumstances permit, you should discuss your predicament with a supervisor or colleague before acting.) In less dangerous situations (e.g., when the patient's developing life story becomes more and more improbable), you should point out the inconsistencies you have noted and ask for the patient's help in resolving them. By leaving room for the implication that you could have misunderstood what the patient was saying, you allow the patient to retract false information and save face in the process.

Schizoid Personality

As a psychiatrist, you hope to maintain a professional objectivity at the same time you convey a personal commitment. This commitment is evident not only in what you do, but also in how you do it. It is important both to care and to be seen to care—to communicate by word and deed your respect for your patients, your belief that they can succeed, and the fact that they matter to you. Most patients respond to your commitment with one of their own, but for schizoid patients such a commitment is hard to make.

The central trait in the concept of the schizoid personality is social detachment, so that schizoid individuals rarely seek out confiding relationships—exactly the type of relationship that best serves the process of psychotherapy. The social isolation of schizoid individuals is not due to fear of criticism or rejection (as it is in people with avoidant personalities) but rather seems to reflect a limited capacity for closeness. Because schizoid patients do not become very attached to you, they are less responsive than many other patients to encouragement.

Another prominent trait of schizoid patients is their emotional restriction—something that characterizes both their capacity to experience emotions and their capacity to express them. This makes it harder for you to know what is important to the patient and whether you are on the right track when making an interpretation or giving a suggestion. Although in the long run you can tell whether you are having an impact on the patient's problem by what the patient reports about his or her life outside of psychotherapy, during psychotherapy sessions you often proceed without clues such as change in the patient's facial expression or tone of voice to tell you how the session is going. You should never attempt to "break through the patient's defenses" or give voice to "countertransference feelings" of frustration at the patient's inertness—such hectoring will only wound a person who may know very well what he or she is missing.

Schizoid patients are less emotionally engaged in psychotherapy than patients with other personality types, but they are not impervious to influence. If you can take the long view and if your goals are realistic (e.g., helping the patient get a job in which there is relatively little contact with other people), progress can be made.

Schizotypal Personality

Like schizoid individuals, those with schizotypal personalities avoid close relationships; like paranoid individuals, they are often suspicious. Because I have already discussed some effects of these traits on the process of psychotherapy, I will focus here on two other prominent characteristics of schizotypal patients: their tendency to have ideas of reference and their odd use of language.

An idea of reference is a mistaken thought that an event has specific personal significance. Anyone can have such a thought, but for most people it is a rare occurrence. You may, for example, believe for a moment that people stop talking as you enter a room because they are talking about you. On reflection, however, you conclude that your arrival coincided with a normal lull in conversation and you make nothing more of it. Schizotypal individuals have ideas of reference much more frequently than other people do, and such ideas are not quickly or easily dismissed. A glance from a stranger on a bus or a statement by a television newscaster can make them anxious and contribute to a sense that others have a special (and perhaps malevolent) interest in them.

This type of thinking has an obvious potential to affect the process of psychotherapy. A remark you make to a colleague as you invite the patient into your office, a new photograph of your family on the wall, a wave of your hand while you talk—such things can be interpreted by the patient as having personal relevance. Is the photograph a sign that you want the patient to marry? Was the wave of your hand a gesture of dismissal? As schizotypal patients work these questions out, they can be distracted from what you are saying or can ask for reassurance about something—like a wave of your hand—you may not even have noticed. If the patient does not tell you that he or she has just developed an idea of reference, you may have a clue to its occurrence if the patient becomes unexpectedly silent. At such times, you can ask the patient whether he or she is wondering about the significance of something you said or did, or something he or she has noticed. There is nothing you can do to prevent the patient from having ideas of reference, though their frequency should diminish as the distress that brought the patient into treatment is reduced.

Schizotypal patients use language in an odd way, so that their speech is often circumstantial, stilted, or vague. Circumstantiality affects the process of psychotherapy by slowing conversation down (and sometimes by exasperating you), but it is a way of speaking by no means limited to schizotypal individuals. Stilted or mannered speech (e.g., using a formal phrase such as "One might say" to begin most sentences) can also slow conversation a bit, but neither it nor circumstantiality makes the patient's thoughts difficult to understand. Vagueness is another matter. The speech of schizotypal patients can be so vague and disjointed that you cannot grasp its point even after asking several times for clarification. If that occurs, you should try restating what the patient has said and asking whether that was what he or she meant. This can be a frustrating process, but the patient is trying to communicate as best he or she can and wants to be understood.

The vague speech of schizotypal patients may reflect, in part, an impairment in abstract reasoning [179]. This impairment could reduce not only their ability to make generalizations in what they are saying, but also their ability to grasp the meaning of generalizations in what you are saying. One type of generalization you might use in psychotherapy is a metaphor—a figure of speech in which a phrase that usually designates one thing is used to designate another. Thus, to a patient frustrated by how long it is taking to repair family relationships, you could say, "Remember, Rome wasn't built in a day." Many patients with other personality types would understand the metaphor to mean "these things take time," but a schizotypal patient could fail to see the relevance of the phrase to your conversation. What does Rome or building have to do with the patient's family? Because schizotypal patients have an impairment in abstract thinking, you should keep your remarks simple and concrete.

Another reason schizotypal patients can have trouble understanding what you say is that they have an impairment in the early stages of verbal learning [178]. One aspect of this difficulty is poor short-term retention of things they are told. To help them compensate for this impairment, you should repeat important information. Whereas with other patients it would be sufficient to say, "When you go to Dr. White's office tomorrow, don't forget to tell him about your dizzy spells," with schizotypal patients it might be better to say, "When you go to Dr. White's office tomorrow, tell him about your dizzy spells. Tell Dr. White about your dizzy spells." Patients whose verbal retention is especially poor should be encouraged to write things down.

Antisocial Personality

When paranoid patients lie to you, it is usually because they want to avoid something; when antisocial patients lie to you, it is often because they want to get something. The defensive lying of paranoid patients is motivated by fear that you will take advantage of them; the offensive lying of antisocial patients is motivated by desire to take advantage of you. Although in reality things are not quite as neat as they appear in these statements, it is useful to distinguish between the lying of paranoid patients and that of antisocial patients, if only because they can provoke such different responses in you.

In general, you will believe that paranoid patients are genuinely distressed and your reaction to their lying may be one of disappointment. In contrast, the lies of antisocial patients will often make you angry because they seem to be feigning distress. On occasion, though, the glib deceitfulness of an antisocial patient is so audacious that it evokes a kind of grudging admiration, which is what Hervey Cleckley may have felt for one of his patients who got into trouble every time he obtained a pass to leave the hospital:

Several days after being returned by his family from such an escapade, Chester came to me smiling and at ease. He spoke briefly of his plans for the future and insisted on having [a pass] at once. In support of this request he sought to make the point that he had proved himself trustworthy and reliable under all circumstances. Looking me squarely in the face, he asserted with modest firmness, "You know that I'm *a man of my word.*" He repeated this statement several times and spoke most intelligently and convincingly on his own behalf. When I asked how he pretended to be a man of his word after breaking it so many times, so flagrantly, and so recently, he showed no signs of being confounded. [28, p. 157]

In addition to being deceitful because they want to avoid obligations, gain privileges, or obtain money, antisocial individuals sometimes lie simply to relieve boredom—to make something happen. Like other extraverts, they need stimulation [38, p. 11]. There is little point in expressing your anger at such behavior. In fact, it may be counterproductive if the patient—seeing that he or she has gotten a rise out of you—is tempted to provoke you again. You should be clear and consistent about the patient's obligations in psychotherapy—including truthfulness—and you should be prepared to terminate treatment if the patient lies repeatedly, but you should do these things with as much equanimity as possible. Expressing the anger you feel to antisocial patients may only reveal another of their traits—aggressiveness.

Nothing disrupts the process of psychotherapy more than a patient who threatens violence. Such threats are more likely to occur if you have scolded an antisocial patient or refused a request that he or she has made, but some antisocial patients use intimidation because they lack the interpersonal skills to get what they want in any other way. Whatever the trigger, the antisocial patient's threshold for aggressiveness is lowered by alcohol [127]. Unless it is an emergency, you should not attempt psychotherapy with any patient—especially an antisocial one—who is intoxicated.

The best way to deal with threats of violence is to prevent them. Antisocial patients are less likely to be aggressive if they understand that you take them seriously, even though you cannot do everything they ask. When patients threaten violence, you can decrease its likelihood by remaining composed and firm. Although this is difficult to do, it usually helps patients restrain themselves:

If the therapist attempts to minimize aggression by vacillating and conciliating, the patient seizes control of the therapy and does in fact dominate the relationship in a bullying kind of way. If the therapist attempts to control aggression by smothering the patient with kindness and reassurance, the patient will likely play the passive role and wait for the therapist to treat him and cure him. . . . [Aggression] must be handled as directly and reasonably as any other symptom, and the therapist who conveys a feeling of confidence and stability is the one who will help the patient most. It would be unrealistic to say that there are not real dangers in the situation, but nothing will cause the patient to lose control faster than loss of control in the therapist. [24, p. 273]

Although threats of violence are the most disruptive manifestation of aggressiveness by antisocial patients, it can also be seen in other forms of interpersonal pressure, including flirtatiousness and requests for money. Here, too, you should strive for equanimity—or at least the appearance of it—as you remind the patient of the limits of a psychotherapeutic relationship.

Borderline Personality

Beginning psychiatry residents sometimes approach the treatment of borderline patients with feelings of incompetence and anxiety. The first of these feelings may emerge as you discover that a great deal has been written about such treatment. How can you hope to undertake psychotherapy with borderline patients until you have read at least some of the literature on the subject? Your sense of inadequacy may only increase as you realize that many of the relevant articles and books have been written by psychoanalysts who use recondite concepts (e.g., projective identification) to explain why borderline patients think, feel, and act as they do. Under the circumstances, you might well conclude that considerable study and specialized training are needed to care for borderline patients and that you are not prepared for the task. Such a conclusion would be unfortunate, because borderline patients can be among the most rewarding of all to treat, even for neophytes.

I believe that, with proper supervision, many beginners are capable of using psychotherapy effectively with borderline patients. If, after a glance at the psychoanalytic literature, you feel incompetent to do so, take heart from the words of Jerome Kroll:

> There are no special procedures, techniques, or secrets which hold exclusively for the therapy of borderlines. The therapy of borderline patients follows the general principles of psychotherapy. One of the basic principles of all therapy is that it be tailored to the clinical state and strengths and needs of the patient. Therefore, the therapy of borderlines will consist of applying general principles of psychotherapy to the specific problems raised by the clinical presentation and situation of the borderline patient. This includes an ongoing assessment of how the characteristically borderline features of the patient have an impact upon and, to some extent, shape the evolving mental and emotional state of the therapist and the process of therapy itself. [103, p. 104]

Two "characteristically borderline features" that affect the process of psychotherapy are a difficulty in sustaining relationships and a low threshold for self-injurious behavior. Even if you believe that, with appropriate supervision, you will be competent to treat borderline patients in general, you may find yourself anxious at the prospect of treating a particular borderline patient because you have already heard about the tribulations that the patient has caused previous psychotherapists.

The trouble borderline patients have in forming stable relationships is due in part to their emotional lability and impulsivity. I will consider the effect of the former trait on the psychotherapeutic relationship when I discuss the histrionic personality, but suffice it to say for now that it is difficult to keep any relationship on an even keel when the other person's mood and behavior are erratic.

Another characteristic of borderline patients that makes for unstable relationships is their tendency to idealize, then denigrate, other people. This tendency, which has been conceptualized in the psychoanalytic literature as a manifestation of the unconscious defense mechanism of *splitting* [94, pp. 29–30], can unexpectedly interrupt the process of psychotherapy. In the initial stages of treatment, borderline patients may regard you as the only person who is understanding enough, trustworthy enough, and constant enough to help them feel good about themselves:

> *Patient:* When I see my parents I get so, so. . . .
> *Psychiatrist:* Angry?
> *Patient:* Yes! I get angry—angry enough to cry.
> *Psychiatrist:* Because they liked your brother better?
> *Patient:* Because they liked my brother better. That's exactly right. Why can't they understand how much it hurt me? You're the only one who understands.

When, inevitably, you fail to live up to the patient's unrealistic expectations, you may be seen as insensitive and uncaring:

> *Psychiatrist:* How was your visit with your parents?
> *Patient:* I don't want to talk about it.
> *Psychiatrist:* Last time, when we discussed your relationship with your parents, we agreed that visiting them might help you clarify some of your feelings. Did it help?
> *Patient:* I don't want to talk about it.
> *Psychiatrist:* Well, perhaps you could tell me why you don't want to talk about it.
> *Patient:* How can you ask me that? You don't understand anything!

The degree to which a borderline patient idealizes or denigrates you may have less to do with your actual qualities than with what the patient desires or fears in a relationship. You may, indeed, be intelligent and insightful, but try to resist the temptation to believe, as the patient does for the moment, that you are the only person capable of helping.

You can diminish the possibility of being denigrated by a borderline patient if you are cautious about supplying words when the patient seems at a loss for them. Sometimes, of course, you will do it and be right (as the psychiatrist was in the first example above), but borderline patients can be hypercritical if you are wrong. Rather than completing sentences for borderline patients, you should encourage them to do so for themselves. This reinforces the idea that being understood depends not on having a magical relationship but on clearly communicating thoughts and feelings:

> *Patient:* When I see my parents I get so, so. . . .
> *Psychiatrist:* Yes. . . .
> *Patient:* So. . . .
> *Psychiatrist:* You get so. . . .
> *Patient:* I don't know. . . . I get angry and sad at the same time, but I love them, too. It's very confusing.

A second characteristic of borderline patients that can affect the process of psychotherapy is their low threshold for self-injurious behavior. Such behavior can take a variety of forms and have a variety of aims. Thus, for example, borderline patients can burn their skin with cigarettes or slice it with razor blades to override a dysphoric mood or to punish themselves; they can take what they know to be a nonlethal overdose of medication to punish someone else (perhaps their psychiatrist) or to bind that person closer to them; and sometimes borderline patients can attempt suicide because they think they have been abandoned or because they have a major depression and are in a hopeless and self-blaming mood. The self-injurious behavior is often impulsive and is more likely to occur if the patient has failed in some way or feels misunderstood or rejected.

Even experienced psychiatrists can find it difficult to choose a course of action when borderline patients threaten self-injury [69, pp. 91–100]. Sometimes this difficulty is due to a conflict between treatment goals. If one goal is to help the patient become more self-reliant, you may think it best to maintain the usual schedule of psychotherapy sessions and to tell the patient to go to an emergency room if self-injury seems imminent. If another goal is to reduce the risk of suicide during a crisis, you may think it best to increase the frequency of sessions or to hospitalize the patient until the crisis is resolved. The course of action you choose will depend to some extent on how well you know the patient, to some extent on your own personality, and, I hope, to a great extent on what your psychotherapy supervisor recommends.

How well you know the patient is a most important variable in judging what is best. Other things being equal, your intervention should be more protective with a patient you have just met than with one you have treated for a year and whose threats of self-injury you know to be expressions of distress rather than statements of intent. Your own personality will also affect the course of action you choose. If you tend to pessimism, you will probably take fewer risks than if you are sanguine by nature. The potential effect of your personality on the choices you make is something you should be able to discuss with your psychotherapy supervisor. In such discussions the supervisor must treat you not as a patient yourself but as a junior colleague who needs advice on a matter of practice. What you want most from your supervisor when a borderline patient threatens self-injury is the opportunity to discuss what to do next, how that intervention relates to your overall plan of treatment, and what you should do if the intervention fails. Whatever you decide, you should document the reasoning behind your choice in the patient's chart.

Try to retain your composure when a borderline patient threatens self-injury. As with an antisocial patient who threatens violence, the calmer you are, the calmer the patient will be. Helping a borderline patient through a crisis and finding a way to minimize or avoid similar crises in the future can be trying experiences for any psychotherapist—but also among the most rewarding.

Histrionic Personality

Although histrionic patients tend to behave in a dramatic, attention-seeking way (e.g., injuring themselves, acting seduc-

tively), such behavior is less likely to affect the process of psychotherapy on a session-by-session basis than are two other
traits of this personality type: impressionistic thinking and emotional lability.

Histrionic individuals find it difficult to think precisely or
deeply about things. What they know of themselves and others
seems not only vague and superficial but also insubstantial and
evanescent. David Shapiro has described this cognitive style as
an impressionistic one:

> Some people search for things in the world—the compulsive
> person for technical data, the paranoid person, even more
> sharply, for clues—while others, hysterics among them, do
> not search, but are struck by things; and what these people
> see are the immediately striking, vivid, and colorful things in
> life. By the same token, the simple factual details, the less ob-
> vious aspects, the contradictions, and the dry, neutral weights
> and measurements of things tend to be absent from hysteri-
> cal notice. The subjective world that emerges in this process
> is a colorful, exciting one, but it is often lacking in a sense of
> substance and fact. [161, p. 119]

This type of thinking is reflected in speech that can be almost
as vague as that of schizotypal patients, though with a much
more dramatic cast:

Patient: You'll never believe what happened Monday night!
Psychiatrist: Tell me about it.
Patient: I've never been so upset in my whole life!
Psychiatrist: What was upsetting to you?
Patient: The whole thing! Everything! Peter was impossible!
Psychiatrist: What did he do?
Patient: What he always does! And Sandra—you should have
    seen her!
Psychiatrist: What did she do?
Patient: She was just as bad. Sandra and the other one love to
    get at me.

Psychiatrist: Sandra and Peter?
Patient: No, Sandra and Denise.
Psychiatrist: I'm still not clear what happened Monday night to upset you.
Patient: I felt like killing someone!
Psychiatrist: But what happened to make you feel like that?

In this example, the psychotherapist struggles, as you will, to help a histrionic patient provide more detail and less drama. Your forbearance in this regard should be greater than that of other people the patient knows—and exasperates. As histrionic patients learn to communicate more clearly in psychotherapy, they not only make their treatment more efficient but also diminish a vulnerability to distress in their everyday lives.

The emotional lability of histrionic patients is disruptive to the process of psychotherapy because it can repeatedly force the psychotherapist into a reactive stance. Whatever else you may have been discussing, when a patient suddenly bursts into tears and rebukes you for something you said, the patient's mood and your responsibility for it become the new topics of conversation. And just as quickly as the sadness and anger are expressed, they may be replaced by other emotions (anxiety, excitement, admiration), depending on your subsequent remarks. This new mood, in its turn, may have to be dealt with, and the carefully considered series of observations and interpretations you had hoped to make at the start of the session must be postponed until another time.

However much nature and nurture contribute to the emotional lability of histrionic individuals [166, pp. 100–105], what triggers a mood change during a psychotherapy session is often your failure to meet the patient's expectations. Sometimes the expectations are clear—and clearly inappropriate; other times they are so subtly expressed that you are unaware of their existence. As Mardi Horowitz noted, the role the histrionic patient is playing at the moment, whether "a sexy star, a wounded hero, or a worthy invalid," is designed to evoke a complementary role —

"interested suitor, devoted rescuer, or responsible caretaker" [86, p. 96]—from the other person in the relationship. If that other person (in this case, you) responds appropriately, the patient's emotions will be positive; if not, they will be negative.

When an emotional storm occurs during a psychotherapy session, you can help the patient by remaining calm, even if this leads to an accusation that you are insensitive and uncaring. (Histrionic patients and borderline patients have many traits in common, so the interventions appropriate for one personality type are appropriate for the other.) Encourage the patient to explain why he or she became upset, clarify any misunderstandings the patient may have had about your remarks, apologize if you have made an error, and (perhaps) link what has just occurred with similar episodes in the past. Histrionic and borderline patients who are suffering rightly expect their psychiatrists to comfort them, but that comforting must be verbal, not physical; professional, not personal.

Narcissistic Personality

Two traits of narcissistic patients that can affect the process of psychotherapy are their superior self-attitude and their feeling of entitlement. Although both can be considered aspects of grandiosity, they have different consequences for the psychotherapeutic relationship.

A narcissistic patient's superior self-attitude is accompanied by an expectation of praise or admiration. Psychiatrists generally look for opportunities to commend patients for their accomplishments, but narcissistic individuals expect more than occasional commendation—they expect frequent and explicit recognition of what they believe to be their special qualities. If those qualities are insufficiently appreciated, narcissistic patients can become angry—as in the following example:

Patient: No one at the office understands how hard I work or what I do for them. No wonder I'm depressed.
Psychiatrist: What would they do if they did understand?

Patient: They'd promote me, that's what!

Psychiatrist: Is there anything you could do to increase the chance of being promoted?

Patient: I could do? I could do? You don't understand—I'm already doing as much I can! You're just like them—you don't see it.

For all their sense of superiority, many narcissistic patients are easily wounded, and such patients can request psychotherapy because they have become demoralized. In the short run, they need help rebuilding their self-confidence and self-esteem. As you express your understanding of their disappointments and as they tell you of past accomplishments, their morale tends to improve and they may leave treatment—feeling better, but with the same vulnerabilities. If there is to be improvement in the long run, you should try to help narcissistic patients understand that many of their expectations are unrealistic and that they will be happier if they can be more sensitive to the opinions and emotions of others [125, pp. 421–24].

Just how unrealistic and insensitive narcissistic patients can be is seen in their feeling of entitlement. Many such patients assume that you will speak with them whenever they telephone, that you will schedule appointments at very short notice, and that clinic staff will assist them immediately, even if other patients have priority. These feelings of entitlement may also include the belief that someone as important or deserving as the patient should be treated by a senior psychiatrist rather than a junior one.

When narcissistic patients act in an entitled way, you should first remind them of the context of treatment. (You do not, for example, answer the telephone when you are with another patient or attending a lecture, unless it is an emergency.) If the patient's behavior continues despite such reminders, you should point out how unrealistic it is and—if you have examples—how such behavior has been a problem for the patient in the past. If that approach fails, or if the patient repeatedly disparages your efforts or credentials, you should offer to help the patient find another psychotherapist, for you cannot be effective if you are always on the defensive.

Avoidant Personality

If patients in psychotherapy are to improve, they must reveal things about themselves and change certain behaviors. Because avoidant patients are fearful of criticism and reluctant to take risks, they find these requirements anxiety-provoking. During psychotherapy with avoidant patients, then, your support and encouragement should be frequent and explicit.

Patients often begin psychotherapy without knowing what to expect from the psychotherapist or what the psychotherapist expects from them. For this reason, you should explain at some time during the first several sessions what the roles of patient and psychotherapist involve. (See also chapter 3.) This "role-induction" process [44, pp. 150–52] may be especially helpful for avoidant patients, who are fearful of being criticized for what they say or do. You can diminish this fear to some extent by pointing out the difference between an observation and a criticism. You can say, for example, that you are not finding fault when you comment on how the patient thinks, feels, or acts but rather calling attention to something that may be a problem. Further, during the initial stages of psychotherapy it is often helpful to preface certain comments with a reminder such as "What I'm going to say now is an observation, not a criticism." This type of reassurance is sometimes necessary well into the course of treatment for avoidant patients because their fear of criticism is difficult to extinguish.

A fear of criticism explains, in part, why avoidant patients are reluctant to take risks—especially the risk of changing their behavior in social situations. Group psychotherapy has a potential advantage over individual psychotherapy in this regard because social interaction is a condition of treatment. When patients with avoidant personalities were treated with group psychotherapy by Lynn Alden and her colleagues, the first factor the patients cited as helpful was the opportunity to meet others who had similar problems [2]. A group experience can reduce the sense of isolation avoidant patients feel and can inspire them to take risks if they see that others in the group are doing so and succeeding. Although individual psychotherapy cannot offer these benefits, it can provide the other two things Alden's patients found useful:

> The second factor nominated was the specific analysis of the individual's social activities and behaviors. Most of these avoidant individuals tended to attribute their avoidance and isolation to some vague, ill-defined, innate, personal inadequacy. The social analysis reframed the problem in terms of specific social activities or behaviors to be enacted in specific social situations, thus making the problem a more manageable one. . . . The third factor identified by these clients was the setting of specific weekly social targets and the encouragement to follow through on these targets. Overall, these elements can be seen as a cognitive reframing of the social avoidance and cognitive and behavioral exposure to fearful situations. [p. 763]

In one regard, individual psychotherapy has a potential advantage over group psychotherapy for avoidant patients, at least at the start, because it may be easier for such patients to reveal things about themselves in a private setting. Whatever the setting, helping avoidant patients reframe their problems and desensitizing them to anxiety-provoking situations should be central to the psychotherapeutic plan.

Dependent Personality

Dependent individuals, even intelligent and accomplished ones, surrender the direction of their lives to other people. Although such individuals usually rely on parents or spouses to take initiatives and make decisions, they can also expect psychotherapists to assume those responsibilities. Dependent patients want more than advice from you: they want to be told exactly what to do, not only about dilemmas (e.g., "Should I put my father in a nursing home?") but also about everyday matters (e.g., "Should

I buy a car with two doors or four?"). Until someone tells them what to do, dependent patients are passive—sometimes to the point of paralysis. Although they agree that passivity is a problem, many return session after session expecting you to make decisions for them. And even when you do, they may need repeated encouragement and reassurance to follow through on what was decided.

Many dependent patients take more initiative as they gain insight into the cost of their passivity (e.g., that it angers others), but some cannot translate insight into action. In these latter cases, you should consider adopting a behavioral approach, praising the patient only when he or she has made a choice or taken an initiative and refusing to make any but the most urgent decisions. If you follow such a course, you must justify it to the patient, who is likely to be upset. One way to begin that justification is to say that you will help the patient analyze what goes into making a particular decision, but that making the decision is the patient's responsibility. If you assume that responsibility, you will diminish the patient's distress in the short run but increase his or her dependence and unhappiness in the long run. Your refusal to direct the patient's life is not a refusal of your obligations as a psychiatrist but rather a way of meeting them—an approach you adopt "out of respect for the patient's right to develop" [186, 2:1171].

Another trait of dependent patients that affects the process of psychotherapy is their reluctance to disagree. Although in some cases this reflects their passivity, in others it seems better explained by a fear of alienating someone on whom they are dependent. When patients do not voice their disagreement with something you have said, they deprive you of an opportunity to make an observation more accurate, an interpretation more apt, or a suggestion more productive. A patient who agrees with everything you say may be doing so for reasons other than your brilliance.

You can help patients—dependent or not—voice their disagreements by making many of your observations, interpretations, and suggestions in a tentative manner. This is certainly the best approach early in treatment, when you still have a great deal to learn about patients. A tentative stance (e.g., "It sounds as if you're angry with your brother. Is that correct?") both makes it easier for patients to contradict you and reinforces the idea that they should be active participants in their psychotherapy.

Obsessive-Compulsive Personality

Histrionic individuals neglect details; obsessive-compulsive individuals are preoccupied with them. This preoccupation can make psychotherapy with obsessive-compulsive patients frustrating if you try to point out the forest while they are still counting the trees:

> *Patient:* . . . so I got angry with him. He didn't follow company policy. He knew very well what he was supposed to do and he tried to cut corners. I had to cover for him and I couldn't do my own work.
>
> *Psychiatrist:* As we've seen before, you got angry because someone didn't follow the rules.
>
> *Patient:* The reason we have a policy is so that everyone knows who's supposed to do what. He took advantage of me once before—because he knows I'm a responsible person.
>
> *Psychiatrist:* Were you angry then?
>
> *Patient:* Yes, I was. The situation was different then because we were working on the same project at the same time. We shared an office and he took a lot of breaks to smoke or have coffee—that sort of thing. But we were expected to get the work out, and the only way that was going to happen was if I did more than my share.
>
> *Psychiatrist:* So you were angry because he didn't follow the rules.
>
> *Patient:* He wouldn't just go out for five minutes—sometimes he'd be gone for ten or fifteen minutes. When he came back, he'd just smile and sit down—he'd never apologize for being away from his desk for so long. I didn't say anything about it at the time because I didn't want to have a confrontation, but I probably should have.

Psychiatrist: So he didn't follow the rules then and he hasn't followed the rules now.

Patient: If he had worked hard when he was at his desk it might have been different. . . .

This preoccupation with details makes it difficult for obsessive-compulsive patients to grasp general points—points such as how their rigidity strains their relationships or how their perfectionism undermines their efficiency. As Leon Salzman noted, "Since the obsessional wants to be precise and clear he introduces more and more qualifications in his presentation to be certain the matter is presented in its fullest form. This adds confusion to the process and, instead of clarifying, tends only to obfuscate the issues" [152, p. 34]. You will have to be persistent in helping obsessive-compulsive patients move from the specific to the general, but the effort is rewarded when they come to understand the vulnerability and use that understanding as a basis for change.

Another trait of obsessive-compulsive patients that affects the process of psychotherapy is doubting. Although doubting is not emphasized in the DSM-IV definition of the obsessive-compulsive personality, it is a central theme in the description of the type over time. Doubting makes obsessive-compulsive patients ambivalent, and ambivalence can be paralyzing. An obsessive-compulsive patient usually makes a detailed analysis of relevant factors before making a decision. A number of alternatives are considered in this process, and one is eventually chosen. In some cases, however, the patient immediately begins to doubt that it was the best choice. This provokes a reconsideration of what had been the leading alternative to the original choice, which is then doubted in turn. At this point, the original choice can appear the better one, and on it goes. The resulting paralysis is often very distressing, and patients may drop the matter entirely or make an impulsive decision simply to end their vacillation.

The doubting experienced by obsessive-compulsive patients sometimes leads to a paralysis more severe than that seen with dependent patients. When dependent patients ask you to make a decision for them and you agree because you want to help get things moving, they usually accept your advice without question. When you make a decision for obsessive-compulsive patients in similar circumstances, their doubting often continues as they analyze your advice and vacillate between the alternatives you provide.

One way to help obsessive-compulsive patients reduce their tendency to doubt is by pointing out a paradox: the more they analyze something in the pursuit of certainty, the less certain they become. Although their analytic ability is a strength in many circumstances, sometimes there can be too much of a good thing. If you make this observation, you should be prepared to answer the question, "Then how do I know when to stop analyzing?" Rather than trying to provide patients with a rule (and have them doubt whether it is applicable in all circumstances), you might turn the discussion to an upcoming decision and have them lay out, in advance, what information they need to make a reasonable choice—not a perfect one. In subsequent sessions, you can help them judge whether further analysis is needed and then get a commitment from them to make a choice and stick to it. In this way, they can see whether the outcome of a decision enacted after appropriate consideration is better than one taken impulsively or not at all.

How the Psychotherapist's Personality Affects the Process of Psychotherapy

It is obvious that the personality of the psychotherapist affects the process of psychotherapy, but how it does so is an awkward subject to discuss. For one thing, there seem to be no reports in which the personalities of psychotherapists are described as DSM-IV types, so I cannot use the approach I took in the last section. For another thing, although there are many small studies of individual traits (e.g., spirituality, flexibility, cultural sensitivity) in psychotherapists belonging to various disciplines (e.g., psychiatry, psychology, social work, nursing, substance abuse counseling), the number of such studies is too large and the methodological differences among them too great for me to summarize in an introductory text. What I can do, however, is address a related topic: do psychiatrists need psychotherapy to be competent psychotherapists?

Do Psychiatrists Need Psychotherapy?

The view that psychiatrists need psychotherapy to be competent psychotherapists probably originated with Carl Jung [144], but its locus classicus is found in a 1912 paper by Sigmund Freud:

> [The doctor] must turn his own unconscious like a receptive organ towards the transmitting unconscious of the patient. He must adjust himself to the patient as a telephone receiver is adjusted to the transmitting microphone. Just as the receiver converts back into sound waves the electric oscillations in the telephone line which were set up by sound waves, so the doctor's unconscious is able, from the derivatives of the unconscious which are communicated to him, to reconstruct that unconscious, which has determined the patient's free associations.
>
> But if the doctor is to be in a position to use his unconscious in this way as an instrument in the analysis, he must himself fulfill one psychological condition to a high degree. He may not tolerate any resistances in himself which would hold back from his consciousness what has been perceived by his unconscious; otherwise he would introduce into the analysis a new species of selection and distortion which would be far more detrimental than that resulting from concentration of conscious attention. It is not enough for this that he himself should be an approximately normal person. It may be insisted, rather, that he should have undergone a psychoanalytic purification and have become aware of those complexes of his own which would be apt to interfere with his grasp of what the patient tells him. [50, pp. 115–16]

Although this requirement applied only to psychoanalysts, the dominant role of psychoanalysis in American psychotherapy for much of the last century led many psychiatry residency programs to recommend psychoanalysis or psychodynamic psychotherapy for their students as a matter of course. Over the years, the rationale for treatment was expanded to include such proposed benefits as having an opportunity to observe a senior psychotherapist in action and becoming more sensitive to the experience of being a patient. Despite the waning influence of psychoanalysis in recent decades and despite the cost of long-term treatment (even when reduced for trainees), many psychiatry residencies have continued to encourage personal psychotherapy. Thus, for example, a survey in 1995 that obtained responses from 86 percent of residency programs in the United States and Puerto Rico showed that 42 percent of them recommended psychotherapy for their residents and 1.2 percent required it [33].

It is difficult to know how many psychiatry residents have had psychotherapy purely to become better psychotherapists and how many have had it for the same reasons other patients do. Indeed, it is difficult to know how many residents have had psychotherapy for any reason. There have been surveys of personal psychotherapy among psychiatry residents over the last 50 years, but even the best of them have produced results that cannot be taken as representative of residents as a whole.

Some of the problems encountered in drawing general conclusions from surveys of residents in psychotherapy are illustrated in an excellent study done in 1994 by Daniel Weintraub and his colleagues [181]. The investigators obtained responses from 96 of 119 (80.7%) residents enrolled in three psychiatry residency programs in Baltimore. The rates of psychotherapy were 60 percent (15/25) among residents in Program A, 6 percent (1/17) among residents in Program B, and 20 percent (11/54) among residents in Program C. The investigators thought it possible that these results could be explained by the degree to which the residents were interested in psychodynamic psychotherapy and the degree to which the programs emphasized it. The finding that 70 percent (19/27) of the residents in psychotherapy had started treatment before beginning their residencies was thought to reflect the long-standing nature of their interest in the subject. Although this conclusion is plausible, it is undercut to some extent by the fact that 78 percent (21/27) of the residents in psychotherapy said they had entered treatment for personal reasons, while only 22 percent (6/27) said they had done so for professional reasons (e.g., to improve their therapeutic skills). It seems to me that even if most of the residents in treatment (15/27) were enrolled in the program (A) with the greatest emphasis on psychodynamic psychotherapy, the reason for treatment was more likely to be clinical than educational.

It is not known the extent to which psychiatry residents in general resemble those in Program A, B, or C. One attempt to gain a broader perspective on the rate of—if not the reason for—personal psychotherapy among residents across the country was made in 1994 by Sidney Weissman, who mailed questionnaires to 1,442 PGY-4 residents [182]. Fifty percent of those responding reported current or past psychotherapy, but the response rate was only 20 percent, so it remains unclear how many residents have psychotherapy and why.

Representative data about personal psychotherapy are lacking not only for psychiatry residents but also for practicing psychiatrists. The most recent large-scale survey involving practicing psychiatrists was done by John Norcross and his colleagues and was published in 1988 [131]. These investigators mailed questionnaires to 500 psychiatrists, 500 clinical psychologists, and 500 social workers whose names had been chosen at random from a national register for each profession. Fifty-six questionnaires could not be delivered, and 719 of the remaining 1,444 were returned, so the overall response rate was 50 percent. The response rates by discipline were 34 percent for psychiatrists, 65 percent for psychologists, and 50 percent for social workers. Because nine practitioners had retired, the final sample of 710 psychotherapists consisted of 159 psychiatrists, 314 psychologists, and 237 social workers.

Of the 710 respondents, 509 (71%) reported at least one

course of personal psychotherapy: 67 percent of the psychiatrists, 75 percent of the psychologists, and 72 percent of the social workers. It was quite common for members of all three disciplines to have had more than one course of treatment: for psychiatrists, the mean number was 2.0; for psychologists, 2.4; and for social workers, 2.3. The majority of all respondents (55%) said they had entered psychotherapy primarily for personal reasons (e.g., marital conflict, depression, anxiety), while 10 percent said they had done so for training reasons. The remaining 35 percent said they had undertaken psychotherapy for both personal and professional goals. Ninety-four percent of all respondents reported significant or moderate improvement after treatment.

The 710 psychiatrists, psychologists, and social workers surveyed were also asked to describe any lessons they had learned about psychotherapy from the experience of being patients themselves. Four hundred and thirteen (58%) mentioned at least one such lesson. The most common responses had to do with the importance of warmth and empathy in the psychotherapeutic relationship, the importance of transference and countertransference issues, the need for patience and tolerance on the part of the psychotherapist, and the psychotherapist's use of the self in treatment. To the extent that these responses are representative of psychotherapists in general, we can conclude that personal psychotherapy can be professionally useful. Such a conclusion is, however, based on reports from psychotherapists who entered treatment primarily for clinical reasons, so it might be expected that, if they were better psychotherapists because of their own psychotherapy, at least part of the improvement might be due to the fact that they were less depressed or anxious or (for example) had less stressful marriages.

There is a difference between what effect psychotherapists think personal psychotherapy has on their practices and what effect it can be shown to have. If psychotherapists who have psychotherapy are demonstrably more skillful than those who have not, psychiatry residents might be shortchanging their patients unless they undergo treatment themselves. The decision to have personal psychotherapy is no small matter, not only because of the time and money involved but also because treatment can have negative effects as well as positive ones, even among those who are enthusiastic about becoming psychotherapists. This last point is illustrated in a survey done by Norman and Ann Macaskill of all 27 senior registrars enrolled in British psychotherapy training programs at the time of the study [119]. (Senior registrars are equivalent to fellows in the United States and their psychotherapy training programs are equivalent to fellowships.) Twenty-five of the 27 (93%) returned the questionnaires, and all 25 were in personal psychotherapy. Nine of the senior registrars who responded (38%) reported negative effects from their treatment. The most common such effects were psychological distress, marital or family distress, and loss of enthusiasm for personal psychotherapy. It is unclear why the rate of negative effects in this survey was so much higher than the rate of 8 percent found by Norcross and his colleagues [131], but it should not be surprising that a treatment with the potential to help also has the potential to harm. Even if we assume a low rate of negative effects from psychotherapy, and even if we assume that its costs in time and money can be borne, the question remains: is there any empirical evidence that personal psychotherapy makes one a better psychotherapist?

According to Susan Macran and David A. Shapiro, the answer to that question is, by and large, no [120]. They reached this conclusion after reviewing 14 studies in which the performance of psychotherapists who had undergone psychotherapy was compared to the performance of psychotherapists who had not. Nine of the studies evaluated clinical outcomes for patients treated with psychotherapy, while five assessed the behavior of psychotherapists during treatment sessions. Given the difficulty of doing such studies, it is not surprising that most were small. Clinical outcomes were evaluated by criteria such as the rate at which patients left treatment prematurely [67; 117] and the degree to which patients improved, as judged by their psychotherapists [55; 93]. Within-session behavior was assessed by criteria such as observer ratings of a psychotherapist's ability to display empathy [170] and genuineness [134]. Although Macran and Shapiro found some evidence that personal psychotherapy can have a positive effect on within-session behavior, they found little evidence to support the claim that personal psychotherapy makes one a better psychotherapist.

It should be reassuring to know that most psychiatrists do not need psychotherapy to be competent psychotherapists. Still, how do you know whether *you* need psychotherapy to be a competent psychotherapist? If you are an introspective person, you may have already noticed how your own traits help or hinder you in the treatment of certain types of patients or certain types of problems. You may have discovered, for example, that being perfectionistic or taciturn creates difficulties for you as a psychiatrist. Learning how to minimize the negative effects of such traits is, in the first instance, a matter for supervision. It should be possible in any residency program to have supervision from someone experienced enough to help you deal with trait-related problems as they affect your care of patients without making you a patient yourself. (This topic is also discussed in chapter 4.)

If you are not an introspective person, it may be your supervisor who points out that you are less effective than you might be because of a trait-related problem. The supervisor may notice, for example, that as you describe your interactions with patients, you give the impression that you are passive or cynical. If, on reflection, you think the supervisor is right, you can adjust your practice accordingly—if you think the supervisor is wrong, you can correct the misimpression. These are delicate matters, but if there is goodwill on both sides, the outcome should be positive.

However a trait-related problem is identified, if it continues despite advice from your supervisor, or if you come to see that it also affects your happiness or performance in other important roles (e.g., spouse, parent, colleague), you should consider psychotherapy in the same way that anyone noting such difficulties might.

Your personality will affect how you practice psychiatry, just as it affects how you do everything else. You should be mindful of characteristics that cause you trouble and try to modify or work around them. Still, most awkward moments in psycho-therapy will be due to the patient's traits, not yours. It is good to be introspective, but you should not become paralyzed by self-doubt. An "approximately normal person" can be a very good psychotherapist.

3. The Psychotherapeutic Relationship

In a culture where self-help books, audiotapes, videotapes, and compact discs are widely available and where computer-based psychotherapy programs are in active development, any discussion of the psychotherapeutic relationship must begin with the question *Is effective psychotherapy possible without a psychotherapist?* The answer seems to be that it is, though only for certain types of people with relatively uncomplicated problems.

Psychotherapy without a Psychotherapist

Self-help materials can be described as inspirational, educational, or therapeutic [115]. Although troubled individuals may benefit from all three types, only materials in the last group present a specific, structured program of treatment. Given the context of such treatment, it is not surprising that most therapeutic programs are cognitive-behavioral in nature.

The self-help programs whose efficacy has been studied can be differentiated on the basis of how much contact, if any, there is with a psychotherapist or other treatment facilitator. Michelle Newman and her colleagues describe four types of program: (1) *self-administered treatment,* in which a psychotherapist does only an initial assessment; (2) *predominantly self-help treatment,* in which a psychotherapist does an initial assessment, provides a therapeutic rationale, and checks in with the patient from time to time; (3) *minimal-contact treatment,* in which a psychotherapist is actively involved, though to a lesser degree than in traditional face-to-face psychotherapy; and (4) *predominantly psychotherapist-administered treatment,* in which the self-help material is used as an adjunct to traditional psychotherapy [130]. Only the first of these types—self-administered treatment—can be considered as psychotherapy without a psychotherapist.

Newman and her colleagues reviewed studies of the efficacy of self-help treatments for anxiety disorders: among them, specific phobias (e.g., snakes), panic disorder, generalized anxiety disorder, and obsessive-compulsive disorder. Although self-administered treatment was found helpful for specific phobias, some contact with a psychotherapist may provide increased benefit for a greater number of phobic patients. The same general results were found for the treatment of panic disorder, with the additional proviso that, although predominantly self-help treatment and minimal-contact treatment can be beneficial, predominantly psychotherapist-administered treatment may be necessary for severely agoraphobic patients. There have been few studies of self-help treatment for generalized anxiety disorder, but both predominantly self-help and minimal-contact techniques have shown promise. All four types of self-help programs appear to have some efficacy in the treatment of obsessive-compulsive disorder, but Newman and her colleagues felt that no firm conclusions could be drawn because of the limited number of studies done to date.

The efficacy of self-help treatments for depression has also been investigated, though not as extensively as the efficacy of such treatments for anxiety. Nancy McKendree-Smith and her colleagues reviewed studies of bibliotherapy and computer-administered therapy for depressive symptoms [115]. Several of the bibliotherapy studies recruited participants from the community who scored above a certain level on self-ratings of depression. In such "depressed" individuals, both minimal contact and predominantly psychotherapist-administered bibliotherapy produced symptom reduction. Very few studies of computer-administered therapy for depression have been done, but McKendree-Smith and her colleagues found several in which computerized cognitive-behavioral therapy was helpful, either as a self-administered treatment for outpatients with major or minor depressive disorders or as an adjunct in the treatment of depressed inpatients.

Jennifer Mains and Forrest Scogin reviewed the efficacy of bibliotherapy for smoking and alcohol abuse [121]. Although self-administered bibliotherapy can help reduce these behaviors, in both cases it seems to work best as part of a more comprehensive program.

The less a psychotherapist is involved in treatment, the more the outcome depends on factors associated with the patient. Thus, for example, poor outcomes are more likely when patients have severe symptoms, personality disorders, low levels of education, and a tendency to externalize the cause of their problems [115; 121; 185].

At present, then, self-administered treatment does not seem to be an effective alternative to psychotherapist-administered treatment for most patients with most psychiatric disorders. Even though self-administered treatments have shown some efficacy for mild anxiety and depression, their usefulness has not been studied in many of the conditions for which psychotherapy is either the essential treatment (e.g., personality disorders, eating disorders) or an important component of treatment (e.g., schizophrenia, sexual disorders). Patients with such disorders need more than information about their problems and suggestions how to solve them—they need a relationship in which they can confide in someone they trust, a relationship in which they are understood as individuals with strengths as well as weaknesses, and a relationship in which the other person sustains hope in the face of adversity. Fortunately, beginning psychiatry residents can easily establish such relationships, which probably explains why the medical students described in the next section were able to do so much good.

Psychotherapy by Medical Students

In 1968, E. H. Uhlenhuth and David Duncan published a study from Johns Hopkins that illustrates the fundamental importance of the psychotherapeutic relationship in determining the outcome of psychotherapy [175; 176]. At the time of the study, the senior medical students at Johns Hopkins had psychiatric clerkships lasting nine to ten weeks. Some students were routinely assigned to the outpatient clinic, where each of them conducted weekly hour-long psychotherapy sessions with a new patient who was considered appropriate for such treatment. Immediately following every session, the student met for half an hour with an instructor (almost always a member of the senior faculty) to discuss the case.

Uhlenhuth and Duncan's study assessed the symptomatic change reported by all 128 outpatients treated by the 128 medical students assigned to the clinic during the academic years 1963–1966. The mean age of the patients was 31 and the great majority of them had "neurotic" disorders or personality disorders. The patients were scheduled to meet with their students for at least six sessions, and the mean number of appointments kept was six. Before each session the patients filled out a 65-item checklist that asked how much they had been troubled by a variety of psychological and physiological complaints in the preceding week. At the time of the first appointment, patients complained most of phenomena related to anger and depression. For the 96 patients who attended five or more sessions, analysis of the checklists revealed that, by the end of treatment, 73 (76%) were improved, none were unchanged, and 23 (24%) were worse.

Although this study assessed symptom change over only several weeks, a similar investigation at the University of Chicago demonstrated that many outpatients treated with psychotherapy by supervised senior medical students maintained their improvement over much longer periods [77]. In the Chicago study, almost all the 249 patients had "neurotic" disorders or personality disorders, and most were seen between 11 and 18 times. The patients were not asked to rate their degree of symptomatic change over the course of treatment, but 75 percent of them were judged to be improved by the students and their supervisors. One hundred and thirty-nine patients were sent questionnaires between 6 and 25 months following their last session to ask, among other things, how they felt then in comparison with how they felt at the end of treatment. Of the 111 patients (80%) who returned the questionnaire, 106 answered that question: 54 (51%) rated themselves as better, 39 (37%) as unchanged, and 13

(12%) as worse. In the interval between ending psychotherapy and completing the questionnaire, only 28 (25%) of the 111 patients had obtained additional treatment. Although the investigators did not provide a statistical analysis of the relationship between additional treatment and symptomatic improvement, they noted that there was a "strong tendency" for patients who described themselves as better on follow-up not to have had subsequent care [p. 178].

In both the Chicago study and the Johns Hopkins study, then, many patients improved when treated by medical students who had little knowledge of the theories and techniques of psychotherapy. What is there about patients, psychotherapists, and the therapeutic alliance between them that makes such outcomes possible? In answering this question I will not review the voluminous literature on the characteristics of participants in psychotherapy and the process of treatment; instead I will discuss some qualities of responsive patients, effective psychotherapists, and good therapeutic alliances that I believe are helpful for beginners to understand.

Some Characteristics of Responsive Patients

Most people who request psychotherapy do so because they are thinking, feeling, or acting in ways that are distressing or maladaptive. They often find it hard to resolve their problems because of conflicts (e.g., desire versus duty) or traits (e.g., dependence) that may or may not be within their awareness. Although many troubled people soldier on for a time, they eventually become demoralized and turn to others for help.

The view that demoralization characterizes patients in psychotherapy was first proposed by Jerome Frank, who (with Julia Frank) wrote that such people "are conscious of having failed to meet their own expectations or those of others, or of being unable to cope with some pressing problem. They feel powerless to change the situation or themselves and cannot extricate themselves from their predicament" [44, p. 35]. Frank and his colleague John de Figueiredo define demoralization as a feeling of distress combined with an awareness of subjective incompetence—a state in which people perceive themselves as lacking the capacity to act or speak in ways they consider appropriate to their circumstances [35].

The Franks note that demoralized patients enter treatment with a variety of symptoms:

At one end of the spectrum are complaints directly related to demoralization, such as anxiety and depression. These are both the most common and the most responsive symptoms of patients in psychotherapy. Other dysphoric emotions, such as anger and resentment, also may be present. At the other end of the spectrum are symptoms that clearly are not caused by demoralization but that often have demoralizing consequences, for example, the cognitive deterioration of Alzheimer's disease or the mood swings of manic-depressive illness. Overall, demoralization may be a cause, a consequence, or both, of presenting symptoms, and its relative importance differs from patient to patient. [44, p. 35]

The Franks acknowledge that not every patient in psychotherapy is demoralized. They recognize, for example, that patients with antisocial personalities or alcohol abuse may be in treatment because their behavior demoralizes others and that those with isolated complaints (e.g., phobias) may enter treatment in the absence of ongoing distress [p. 36]. Still, they believe that demoralization characterizes most people who request psychotherapy and that the restoration of morale is an important component of treatment, especially in its early phases. Demoralized patients want leadership and hope, both of which even beginning psychotherapists can provide.

Patients also want to be understood on their own terms, even as they admit their failings. This, too, is something beginners can provide. When patients give voice to thoughts and emotions hitherto unexpressed, and when those thoughts and emotions are validated in some way, they feel better. Part of the relief comes from simple catharsis, from saying aloud what was previously unspoken or from owning up to a shameful act, but part also comes from being understood, which is itself a kind of absolution:

> *Patient:* I was so angry with him that I just let him have it— right there in front of the whole office. The guy is so timid it's nauseating. Why can't he just say what he thinks when I want his opinion? I know I shouldn't have done it, but the pressure was really on and I needed a decision—fast. By the time I was done with him, he was crying and apologizing, which just made me angrier.
>
> *Psychiatrist:* The contract was on the line. Right?
>
> *Patient:* Right.
>
> *Psychiatrist:* So your job was on the line.
>
> *Patient:* Right.
>
> *Psychiatrist:* So you lost your temper.
>
> *Patient:* Yes.
>
> *Psychiatrist:* Anyone in your shoes would have felt the pressure.
>
> *Patient:* Yes, but not everyone would have done what I did.
>
> *Psychiatrist:* Probably not. Did you apologize to him?
>
> *Patient:* No, I went back to my office and took care of business.
>
> *Psychiatrist:* Do you think you should apologize?
>
> *Patient:* Yes, but if I do he'll say it was all his fault and I'll just get angry again.
>
> *Psychiatrist:* Still. . . .
>
> *Patient:* No, you're right. I'll do it. I just wish I wouldn't get so mad at people who can't stand up for themselves.
>
> *Psychiatrist:* Have you always been like that?

Although most patients need more than understanding and the restoration of morale to achieve long-term change, if the former are not provided, the latter is unlikely to occur.

Some Characteristics of Effective Psychotherapists

Beginning psychotherapists can provide the understanding, leadership, and hope that most patients desire. What patients desire, however, might not be what they need. It could be, for example, that an aloof and passive but technically brilliant psychotherapist is more effective than an affable and energetic but less proficient one.

There are two approaches to defining the characteristics of effective psychotherapists: the distillation of clinical experience and the investigation of factors associated with good treatment outcomes. The first approach is illustrated by the reflections of Stanley Greben, who wanted to identify the attributes of successful psychotherapists:

> Those qualities which underlie "being therapeutic" are very much a matter of *character of the therapist,* rather than being a matter of his technique. . . . In all my conversations with people who have been helped by therapists, and this includes many therapists and psychoanalysts themselves, none have said, for example, the good results were achieved by virtue of the correctness and brilliance of the therapist's interpretations. . . . I have never been told: "He had a dazzling way of leaping to the heart of the matter, with explanations which surprised and relieved me." Much more often I would be told, "He turned out to be a decent human being who, I finally came to believe, really cared for me, and for what happened to me." [65, p. 374]

Based on his long experience as a psychotherapist and teacher of psychotherapy (including psychoanalysis), Greben proposed that successful psychotherapists demonstrate:

- empathy and concern
- a caring and protective attitude
- a warm manner
- an ability to arouse hope
- an expectation of improvement
- a refusal to despair
- personal reliability
- friendliness and respectfulness

The second way of defining the characteristics of effective psychotherapists has been to study factors associated with good treatment outcomes. This empirical approach has identified many attributes that can influence success with particular types of patients or in particular clinical situations or using particular psychotherapeutic techniques. Among the factors studied have been the psychotherapist's age, sex, ethnicity, personality, emotional well-being, values, professional background, and experience [17]. Within this body of work there is a long history of attempts to identify those characteristics that are fundamental to success in treatment, whatever the type of patient, clinical situation, or psychotherapeutic technique. Perhaps the best known of these attempts is a series of studies by Charles Truax and his colleagues, who found that a combination of empathy, warmth, and genuineness (authenticity) contributed to positive outcomes [173]. Although there is widespread agreement that these qualities affect the results of treatment, there has been controversy about whether they are as powerful as initially thought [126; 148] and whether the research that identified them was methodologically sound [9; 160; 174]. Still, it is hard to imagine that a psychotherapist lacking empathy could have much insight into a patient's problems (save for straightforward ones such as phobias) or that one lacking in warmth or genuineness could sustain a relationship in which the patient is expected to be candid and trusting.

Although some psychotherapists are naturally more effective than others, all psychotherapists can be mindful of the qualities most helpful to patients. If you are not a very empathic person, you can compensate to some extent by listening carefully to patients and by asking them to describe their experiences fully; if you are not a very warm person, you can maintain eye contact with patients and communicate your understanding of their distress; and if you sometimes want to appear as more than you are, you can remember that the role you have chosen—that of a psychiatrist—is best played modestly.

Some Characteristics of Good Therapeutic Alliances

Over the years, the therapeutic alliance between patients and psychotherapists has been defined and measured in many ways [39; 60; 88; 110; 124]. One of the most straightforward definitions was proposed by Edward Bordin, who wanted to describe the concept in terms that were applicable to all types of psychotherapy [19]. According to Bordin, the therapeutic alliance has three components: (1) an agreement on goals (what changes the patient wishes to make); (2) an agreement on tasks (how those changes are to be accomplished); and (3) the development of bonds. The first two components are cognitive in nature; the last, affective.

The tasks of treatment are determined in part by the type of psychotherapy employed. A phobic patient in psychoanalysis would have the task of free association, while the same patient in behavior therapy would have the task of desensitization. Some tasks, of course, are fundamental to all types of psychotherapy, so that no matter what approach is taken, patients understand that they must be forthright about their problems, and psychotherapists understand that they must explain the reasons for their recommendations. As treatment proceeds, new goals and tasks often arise. Thus, a psychotherapist and a patient who had agreed to meet weekly to discuss the latter's distress over a failing marriage might agree to meet twice a week if a divorce seemed imminent.

The process of agreeing on goals and tasks contributes to the bond that develops between patients and psychotherapists, but that bond depends much more on the interaction of two other factors: the extent to which the participants fulfill the agreements they have made and the extent to which their personalities are compatible. A patient and a psychotherapist may produce a serviceable bond if they meet their commitments even though each has some traits that annoy the other, while a patient and a psychotherapist who sometimes fail in their mutual responsibilities may sustain an effective bond because they are well-matched as individuals.

Patients and psychotherapists make conscious decisions about the goals and tasks of treatment; they do not make conscious decisions about whether they will respect and like one another. Respect and affection develop, if at all, in the context of the emerging relationship, and relationships involve unconscious as well as conscious processes. (The notion that personality traits and unconscious processes are determinants of the bond between patients and psychotherapists raises the topics of transference and countertransference, which I will discuss later in this chapter.)

There is a great deal of empirical support for the claim that a good therapeutic alliance predicts a good treatment outcome [78; 79; 89; 104]. This positive association is not a function of the type of psychotherapy employed, and it is found with cognitive and behavioral, as well as psychodynamic, approaches. The quality of the therapeutic alliance is determined early in the relationship [11; 87], so it is important to get things off to a good start. One way to do this is by preparing patients for psychotherapy during the initial meeting.

Every new patient has ideas about what psychotherapy is and what psychotherapists do. Very often, such ideas are wrong. In this regard, the situation today is much the same as that described forty years ago by Rudolf Hoehn-Saric and his colleagues:

> Because of the diversity and ambiguities of public conceptions of mental illness and psychotherapy, psychiatric patients reach the psychiatrist's office with a wide variety of attitudes and expectations. Only the most sophisticated are perfectly clear about why they are there and what they expect. Less sophisticated patients may have unrealistic expectations for improvement: they may not understand their role in the therapeutic process and may be bewildered by a procedure that differs not only from usual medical treatment but from customary social interactions. [82, p. 267]

In preparing new patients for psychotherapy, then, you should explain how talking about problems can lead to their solution. This explanation must be given in terms the patient can understand and should make reference to the patient's complaints. You should set out what the patient can expect of you and what you expect of the patient. You should be optimistic about the outcome of treatment, even as you anticipate difficulties that may occur. The following is a highly condensed example of what might be said:

> *Psychiatrist:* Why do you think you keep getting into relationships that hurt you?
>
> *Patient:* I don't know. It's like I'm stuck in a pattern and I can't figure out why.
>
> *Psychiatrist:* So what we need to do is discover what keeps the pattern going, and once we do that, you should be able to change it. I'll be asking you a lot of questions about your background, your personality, and the relationships you've had, and that will give us important information. I hope you'll answer the questions frankly.
>
> *Patient:* I'll do my best.
>
> *Psychiatrist:* Good. Once we understand what's causing the problem, we can work to correct it. If I think you're on the wrong track, I'll explain why, and I hope you'll do the same for me. For you to feel better, you'll have to change how you think about yourself or how you act with other people. Changes like that can be hard. In fact, sometimes they can be so hard that you might not want to come in for an appointment. If that happens, please come in anyway—you might make the most progress when you least expect it. I just said that change can be difficult, but I also want you to know that most patients can improve—sometimes a lot—if they try. The fact that you're here is a good sign. Now, any questions about what I've said so far?

There is some empirical support for better outcomes (at least in the short term) when patients get this type of preparation at the start of treatment [27; 82; 108; 168]. Even without such support, however, it is your responsibility to prepare patients for psychotherapy (as you would prepare them for any treatment) and to invite questions about what you have said. As you do this, you will demonstrate your respect for the patient's intelligence and make it clear that psychotherapy is a collaborative effort.

Transference, Countertransference, and Determinants of the Psychotherapeutic Relationship

Transference

The term *transference* was coined by Sigmund Freud to describe a form of resistance in psychoanalysis. The patient, instead of remembering and discussing thoughts and feelings about a person in the past, experiences those thoughts and feelings about the psychoanalyst in the present. The clinical example Freud provided in his initial definition of transference in 1895 illustrates the essence of the concept:

> In one of my patients the origin of a particular hysterical symptom lay in a wish, which she had had many years earlier and had at once relegated to the unconscious, that a man she was talking to at the time might boldly take the initiative and give her a kiss. On one occasion, at the end of a session, a similar wish came up in her about me. She was horrified at it, spent a sleepless night, and at the next session, though she did not refuse to be treated, was quite useless for work. . . . The content of the wish had appeared first of all in the patient's consciousness without any memories of the surrounding circumstances which would have assigned it to a past time. The wish which was present was then . . . linked to my person . . . and as the result of this *mésalliance*—which I describe as a "false connection"—the same affect was provoked which had forced the patient long before to repudiate this forbidden wish. [49, pp. 302–3]

By the middle of the last century, some of Freud's intellectual heirs had greatly expanded the concept of transference. For them, almost every aspect of the patient's relationship with the psychoanalyst was a repetition of past (usually childhood) relationships, and almost every communication—both verbal and nonverbal—was transferential in nature [153]. Because a definition this broad deprived the concept of specificity and obscured what actually happened in the room during treatment, many psychoanalysts refused to accept it. Contemporary psychoanalytic definitions of transference are anchored in Freud's original concept, but they give greater emphasis than he did to the notion that the patient's thoughts, moods, and behaviors are shaped to some extent by what the psychoanalyst does. As Richard Chessick puts it:

> The result of the pressure of [the patient's] internal childhood fantasies is that there is a tendency to reenact them in all interpersonal relationships, always attempting to actualize a derivative representation of an unconscious fantasy. Without being aware of it, the [patient] tries to impose a preconceived situation onto a new situation. . . .
>
> The analyst's behavior or style or countertransference is a stimulus for the patient's unconscious fantasy life that sets off the reaction we call transference. The analyst is given an assigned role to play in the preconceived drama and tremendous pressure is placed on him or her to act and speak in a way consistent with that unconsciously assigned role. [26, p. 95]

Countertransference

Freud wrote much less about countertransference than he did about transference. In fact, he scarcely defined the term *countertransference* at all, save to say that it arose in the psychoanalyst "as a result of the patient's influence on his unconscious feelings" [45, p. 144]. Freud saw countertransference as an impediment to treatment because it distorted the psychoanalyst's understanding of the patient, and he eventually recommended all psychoanalysts be psychoanalyzed to make them aware of the unconscious determinants of their countertransference reactions. (See chapter 2.) Although Freud provided few specifics

about his concept of countertransference, historians of psycho-
analysis such as Joseph Sandler and his colleagues have fleshed
it out:

> It is clear that Freud included in counter-transference more
> than the analyst's transference (in the sense in which he
> used the term) to his patient. While it was true that a patient
> might come to represent a figure of the analyst's past,
> counter-transference might arise simply because of the ana-
> lyst's inability to deal appropriately with those aspects of the
> patient's communications and behaviour which impinged on
> inner problems of his own. Thus if a psychoanalyst had not
> resolved problems connected with his own aggression, for ex-
> ample, he might need to placate his patient whenever he de-
> tected aggressive feelings or thoughts toward him in the pa-
> tient. . . . The "counter" in counter-transference may thus
> indicate a reaction in the analyst which implies a *parallel* to
> the patient's transferences (as in "counterpart") as well being
> a reaction to them (as in "counteract"). [154, p. 84]

In the decades following Freud's description of countertransference as an impediment to treatment, psychoanalytic thinking
on the topic began to change in two ways. First, the definition of
countertransference was expanded, so that some psychoanalysts
came to designate almost all emotional reactions to the patient
as countertransference phenomena. This expanded definition,
unlike the expanded definition of transference noted above,
found wide acceptance in the psychoanalytic community. Second, countertransference was increasingly seen not as an obstacle to understanding patients but as an asset. The rationale
for this latter change was stated in 1950 by Paula Heimann:

> My thesis is that the analyst's emotional response to his patient
> within the analytic situation represents one of the most im-
> portant tools for his work. The analyst's counter-transference
> is an instrument of research into the patient's unconscious.
> The analytic situation has been investigated and described

from many angles, and there is general agreement about its unique character. But my impression is that it has not been sufficiently stressed that it is a *relationship* between two persons. What distinguishes this relationship from others, is not the presence of feelings in one partner, the patient, and their absence in the other, the analyst, but above all the degree of the feelings experienced and the use made of them, these factors being interdependent. The aim of the analyst's own analysis, from this point of view, is not to turn him into a mechanical brain which can produce interpretations on the basis of a purely intellectual procedure, but to enable him, to *sustain* the feelings which are stirred in him, as opposed to discharging them (as does the patient), in order to *subordinate* them to the analytic task. [76, pp. 81–82]

The feelings which were stirred in the psychoanalyst were now seen as resonating with the patient's unconscious wishes and fears—wishes and fears that were as yet unspoken but nonetheless influenced the patient's behavior during the session. Thus, a psychoanalyst who felt annoyed while a patient spoke critically of her mother might subsequently link that feeling to the patient's narcissistic desire for praise. Countertransference was thought to reveal important information not only about the nature of the patient's unconscious feelings but also about the degree of the patient's regression, so that "the more intense and premature the therapist's emotional reaction to the patient, the more threatening it becomes to the therapist's neutrality . . . the more we can think the therapist is in the presence of severe regression in the patient" [95, p. 43].

Although many psychotherapists do not find the psychoanalytic concept of regression useful, they do believe that emotions provoked by a patient's verbal and nonverbal communications can provide hints to the patient's underlying psychological state. (It is, of course, essential to regard such hints *as* hints, rather than facts, lest you fall into the trap of believing that your "gut feelings" are an infallible source of information about the patient—something a psychoanalyst would warn against.)

Just as contemporary students of transference such as Richard Chessick (see above) invoke countertransference to explain what they mean by the concept that interests them, so contemporary students of countertransference such as Glen Gabbard invoke transference to explain what they mean by the concept that interests *them*:

> Today, clinicians of all persuasions generally accept the idea that countertransference can be a useful source of information about the patient. At the same time, the therapist's own subjectivity is involved in the way the patient's behavior is experienced. Hence, there is a movement in the direction of regarding countertransference as a *jointly created* phenomenon that involves contributions from both patient and clinician. The patient draws the therapist into playing a role that reflects the patient's internal world, but the specific dimensions of that role are colored by the therapist's own personality. [52, p. 984]

Determinants of the Psychotherapeutic Relationship

For all that has been written about transference and countertransference, they are not the major determinants of the psychotherapeutic relationship. Other factors are more important, both because they operate earlier in the relationship and because they are more fundamental to it. In my view, those factors are the social roles of patient and psychotherapist, the treatment approach used by the psychotherapist, and the personalities of the patient and the psychotherapist.

To be a patient, a psychotherapist, a parent, a teacher, a soldier, or a priest is to occupy a certain social role. Each role is characterized by a set of attitudes and behaviors that are expected of its occupant. Thus, for example, patients are expected to regard illness as an undesirable state and to cooperate with physicians and others who try to help them get well, while physicians are expected to regard their patients as worthy of help and to refrain from exploiting them. Although most people are quite familiar with the attitudes and behaviors expected of patients in general, those expected of patients in psychotherapy are less familiar, which is why it is important to prepare patients for treatment in the manner described above. In a similar way, although by now you are quite familiar with the attitudes and behaviors expected of physicians in general, those expected of you as a psychotherapist are less familiar, which is why it is important for you to have supervision. All psychotherapeutic relationships are grounded in the social roles of the participants, a fact that becomes especially—sometimes painfully—obvious when the boundaries of those roles are transgressed. (See below for a discussion of the boundaries of the psychotherapeutic relationship.)

A second major factor determining the psychotherapeutic relationship is the treatment approach adopted by the psychotherapist. Do you ask about the patient's fantasies or not? Are you on a first-name basis with the patient or not? Do you use hypnosis or not? Do you ask the patient to sit in a chair or lie on a couch? Do you touch the patient or not? These are more than technical questions; their answers determine whether certain types of thoughts and actions are discouraged, tolerated, or promoted.

Although Sigmund Freud sat behind his reclining patients because he could not stand being stared at for eight hours a day, he also did it to avoid contaminating their transference reactions: "Since, while I am listening to the patient, I, too, give myself over to the current of my unconscious thoughts, I do not wish my expressions of face to give the patient material for interpretations or to influence him in what he tells me. The patient usually regards being made to adopt this position as a hardship and rebels against it. . . . I insist on this procedure, however, for its purpose and result are to prevent the transference from mingling with the patient's associations imperceptibly, to isolate the transference and to allow it to come forward in due course sharply defined as a resistance" [47, p. 134]. This psychoanalytic technique fosters a very different type of relationship between the psychotherapist and the patient than the Gestalt technique developed by Fritz Perls:

In this model, the therapist is available for work with one person . . . at a time. The volunteer client takes the "hot seat" facing the therapist, sometimes in the center of the group and sometimes in the circle of group members. While the therapist and client explore whatever phenomena emerge in their interaction, the rest of the group members remain silent and are spectators, not unlike the Greek choruses who replied to or commented on the dramatic action in the play. Although limited, the chorus performed an essential function, as does the group in Gestalt therapy. At certain points the group may be called into action by the therapist, but usually this is done in a structured way to further the client's work. . . .

The controlling factor in the client's interaction with the group members is the therapist's intention to keep the focus on the client and to encourage that person to take responsibility for his or her own experience. [99, pp. 105–6]

The treatment approach you adopt provides a script for you and the patient to follow. It decides, to a greater or lesser degree, how the two of you interact, which words you use when speaking to one another, and what constitutes a good performance. The social roles of the psychotherapist and the patient determine the general character of their relationship; the treatment approach gives those roles more definition.

Personality is the third major factor determining the nature of the psychotherapeutic relationship. The less doctrinaire your treatment approach, the more your personality and that of your patient shape the expression of your social roles and the affective component of the therapeutic alliance. Even if you stick to the script of a single therapeutic method, your relationship with patients will differ to the extent that they are dependent or independent, trusting or suspicious, impertinent or respectful. In the same way, their response to you will vary to the degree that you are controlling or permissive, jocular or solemn, predictable or erratic.

Every now and then a patient or a psychotherapist does something out of character and their relationship suffers. One reason for such occurrences is the displacement of feelings from another relationship or situation—not in the sense of transference or countertransference (in the Freudian meaning of the latter term), but in the sense that you might be irritable with Patient A because ten minutes earlier you were insulted by Patient B. If this happens, an apology from the offending party should set matters right.

Another reason that patients or psychotherapists sometimes act out of character is that they are intoxicated or have developed an illness such as depression or mania. If a patient is intoxicated, you should abort the session with a reminder that psychotherapy requires concentration and reflection. Intoxication in a psychotherapist is more serious than intoxication in a patient. A psychotherapist who is intoxicated ipso facto has poor judgment. That psychotherapist also has difficulty concentrating and therefore difficulty thinking through complicated issues—exactly the type of thinking a patient has every right to expect. If you attempt to practice psychotherapy while intoxicated, you violate the patient's trust. Rather than risk harm to the patient, you must cancel the session. If you are intoxicated more than once, you must suspend your practice and obtain treatment.

When patients develop severe depression or mania, the cause of their uncharacteristic behavior is obvious; when the affective disorder is mild, however, it might take several sessions for you to realize what is happening. You can make the diagnosis more quickly if you do a mental status examination whenever there is an unexpected change in a patient's mood, thinking, or behavior, especially if it persists from session to session. Stepping back from the flow of psychotherapy can help you see that, although Patient A *might* be irritable because she is ambivalent about what you are asking her to do or Patient B *might* be taciturn because he is having a transference reaction, the correct explanation for their uncharacteristic behavior is that each has developed an affective disorder.

When psychotherapists become severely depressed, they usually feel ill, doubt their abilities, have difficulty concentrating, and lose the drive to work. For these reasons, they often stop seeing patients and enter treatment, either on their own—especially if they have been depressed in the past and recognize a relapse—or with encouragement from family members or colleagues. When psychotherapists become severely manic, however, they usually do not see themselves as ill and they resist the advice of relatives and colleagues to consult a psychiatrist, even if they have been manic before. Like other people with severe mania, they usually have great confidence in their abilities despite the fact that their thinking is disorganized, and they can do a great deal of harm to themselves and others—including their patients—if they are irritable or hypersexual.

Although psychotherapists with mild affective disorders often continue to work, their illness can damage their relationship with their patients. If a depressed psychotherapist is apathetic, for example, a patient who needs encouragement may not get it. And if a hypomanic psychotherapist is condescending, a patient with low self-esteem may feel even more debased. If you ever wonder whether you have an affective disorder, or if a relative or colleague raises the question, you owe it to your patients, your family, and yourself to take the matter seriously.

Finally, patients and psychotherapists can act out of character because they are having transference and countertransference reactions, respectively. (Here I am using *countertransference* in the Freudian sense.) When this occurs, the emotions expressed are intense and inappropriate to the situation. If you suspect a transference or countertransference reaction, discuss your observations with your psychotherapy supervisor, who should be able help you identify the phenomenon and deal with it.

The Boundaries of the Psychotherapeutic Relationship

Although you may have affectionate—even amorous—feelings for your patients, you must not encourage them to become your lovers. Although you use the psychotherapeutic relationship to help patients overcome their problems, you must not use it to help overcome your own. And although you gain monetarily from the care you provide, you must not exploit your patients financially. If you do these things, you violate the boundaries of the psychotherapeutic relationship and the trust your patients have placed in you.

People become psychotherapists to help others, not to harm them, so why do some psychotherapists act unethically? One reason is that their judgment is impaired by intoxication or a disorder such as depression or mania. When this occurs, the affected psychotherapist can show poor judgment about many things in both professional and nonprofessional relationships. (In the rare case of psychotherapists with paraphilic disorders, the impairment of judgment is much more restricted in scope.) Another reason psychotherapists can act unethically is that, despite the values instilled by their professional education—and sometimes despite their personal psychotherapy—they yield to antisocial, borderline, histrionic, narcissistic, or dependent traits when their nonprofessional relationships are unsatisfactory or when (as sometimes occurs) a patient entices them. A final reason is that psychotherapists, whatever their personalities, can deceive themselves into thinking that they are acting in their patients' interest rather than their own [51]. Such self-deceptions may be especially common in sexual misconduct.

Sexual Misconduct

According to Robert Simon, there is a fairly typical sequence of events in sexual misconduct by psychotherapists [164]. The sequence may begin when the psychotherapist and the patient start to address one another by their first names. After that, their sessions become increasingly social in nature and the psychotherapist reveals more and more about his or her own feelings and interests. In due course the sessions, which used to end verbally, terminate with a handshake and then with a hug. Eventually, sessions are scheduled for the end of the day, after which the couple begin to have dinner with each other and, perhaps, see a movie together. Hand-holding, kissing, and intercourse follow in their turns. Simon identifies the time "between the chair and the door" as an especially dangerous transition in this sequence [165], but it is easy to understand how each transition could lower the threshold for the following one.

Thomas Gutheil and Glen Gabbard described this process as a "slippery slope" [71; 72]. In doing so, they indicated both the gradual nature of the descent into misconduct and the difficulty a psychotherapist can have in stopping it. Jerome Kroll criticizes the notion of a slippery slope on empirical and conceptual grounds [102]. Kroll wants to know, for example, how often psychotherapists and patients who address each other by their first names actually proceed to sexual intercourse. He insists that the earliest acts in the sequence described by Simon—the use of first names and limited self-disclosure by psychotherapists—are perfectly acceptable techniques in certain treatment methods and therefore do not ipso facto represent crossings of the boundary between a professional and a personal relationship. Kroll identifies the slippery-slope argument as a post hoc one— a point also made by Ofer Zur and Arnold Lazarus: "To assert that self-disclosure, a hug, a home visit, or accepting a gift are actions likely to lead to sex is like saying that doctors' visits cause death because most people see a doctor before they die" [190, p. 9].

Gutheil, Gabbard, and Simon responded to such criticisms by (among other things) reiterating their acknowledgment that techniques appropriate in one treatment method might not be appropriate in another [51; 73; 163]. Thus, for example, "a behavior therapist assisting an agoraphobic patient through use of in vivo exposure may drive the patient to a shopping mall to encounter the feared situation. A clinician engaged in psychoanalytic psychotherapy would be in serious need of supervision if similar activities were going on. Even within psychodynamic therapy, however, the appropriate frame varies from patient to patient. Certain patients require greater degrees of verbal activity or therapeutic self-disclosure for them to feel engaged in a treatment process. Also, some therapists may have a more self-revelatory style than others" [71, pp. 411–12]. Gutheil, Gabbard, and Simon allow for variations in treatment technique and personal style, but their experience evaluating and treating psychotherapists who commit sexual misconduct leads them to conclude that the unethical behavior often begins with a series of apparently harmless acts.

How Many Psychotherapists Find Their Patients Attractive? It is reasonable to assume that the number of psychotherapists who find their patients sexually attractive is much greater than the number who commit sexual misconduct. To my knowledge, only one study has tested that assumption. The study was published in 1986 by Kenneth Pope and his colleagues, who tried to ascertain how many psychologists found their patients attractive and what they found attractive about them [139]. The investigators sent an anonymous questionnaire to 500 male and 500 female psychologists randomly selected from the 4,356 members of the American Psychological Association's division for psychologists in private practice. Of the 1,000 potential respondents, 585 (58.5%) returned the questionnaire, and of these, 339 (57.9%) were men and 246 (42.1%) were women. Almost half (48.9%) of the respondents were between the ages of 30 and 45; 39.0 percent were between 46 and 60; and 12.1 percent were over 60. As a group, they averaged 16.9 years of professional experience.

Five hundred and eight of the 585 respondents (86.8%) reported being attracted to at least one patient, with 322 (94.9%) of the men and 186 (75.6%) of the women acknowledging such feelings. When asked in an open-ended question what it was about their patients they had found attractive, the respondents answered with 997 descriptive terms, which the investigators sorted into 19 categories. The largest category (296 responses) was physical attractiveness, which included terms such as *beautiful* and *athletic*. The next largest category (124 responses) was intellectual attractiveness, which included terms such as *intelligent* and *articulate*. The third-largest (88 responses) was sexual attractiveness, which not only included terms such as *sexy* but also notations that sexual material was discussed during psychotherapy, while the fourth-largest (85 responses) had to do with the patient's vulnerabilities, as indicated by terms such as *childlike* and *sensitive*.

Although the vast majority of psychologists surveyed had

found some patients attractive for one reason or another, 93.5 percent said they had never been sexually intimate with their patients. (What constituted sexual intimacy was not defined in the paper.) Among the 6.5 percent of respondents who acknowledged sexual intimacy with patients, the rate was higher among men (9.4%) than women (2.5%). Most respondents (57.0%) who were sexually attracted to patients sought supervision or consultation about their feelings—a practice that was more common among younger psychologists than older ones but equally common among males and females.

The psychologists who reported having been attracted to patients without becoming sexually involved gave a variety of reasons for their abstinence. The open-ended question that assessed this topic generated 1,091 responses, which the investigators sorted into 14 categories. The largest category (289 responses) was that sexual involvement with patients was unethical. The next largest were that it was countertherapeutic or exploitative (251 responses), unprofessional (134 responses), or against the respondent's personal values (133 responses).

Although the study by Pope and his colleagues is a valuable one, it faces two methodological questions that confront all self-report surveys: (1) Is the sample representative? and (2) Are the responses valid? The latter question may be especially important when the topic of the survey is a stigmatized behavior such as sexual misconduct or substance abuse. One indication of the potential gap between what people report they do and what they actually do can be found in a 1992 survey sent by John Lamont and Christel Woodward to all 792 members of the Society of Obstetricians and Gynaecologists of Canada [106]. Six hundred and eighteen (78.0%) members responded, and of these, 497 (80.4%) were male and 121 (19.6%) were female. The average age of the respondents was 47.3 years and their average time in practice was 16.8 years. Of this sample, 3 percent of the males and 1 percent of the females acknowledged sexual involvement (according to the respondent's own definition of that phrase) with someone who was a patient at the time. In contrast, 17 percent of females and 8 percent of males reported knowing that a colleague in obstetrics and gynecology had been involved with a current patient. Although it is possible that the latter figures could overestimate the frequency of sexual misconduct by Canadian obstetricians and gynecologists if several respondents were aware of the same colleague's behavior, my point here is that the actual rate of sexual misconduct in any group is almost certainly higher than the rate derived from self-reports.

Methodological issues notwithstanding, anonymous self-report surveys have been the most common way of estimating the frequency of sexual misconduct by physicians in general, by practicing psychiatrists, and by psychiatry residents. What do such surveys reveal?

How Common Is Sexual Misconduct by Physicians in General? If the Hippocratic Oath is any indication, sexual misconduct by physicians has been a problem for thousands of years. In the traditional version of the Oath, physicians swear to "come for the benefit of the sick, remaining free of all intentional injustice, of all mischief and in particular of sexual relations with both female and male persons, be they free or slave" [37, p. 3]. Despite this and similar prohibitions over the centuries, and despite the principle of *primum non nocere ("first, do no harm")*, physicians have continued to engage in sexual misconduct.

Table 2 summarizes the results of eight surveys of physicians in various specialties about their sexual involvement with current or former patients. Although the studies differ in how they defined and asked about sexual involvement, in the size and diversity of the groups they sampled, and in the response rates they achieved, all of them discovered some physicians who were willing to acknowledge (and in some cases to defend as therapeutic) behaviors that ranged from touching for the purpose of sexual arousal to intercourse. The rates of sexual involvement differed from study to study for a given specialty (e.g., 3 to 10 percent for obstetrics and gynecology), but considering all of the studies, the rates were roughly comparable from one specialty to another. In the six surveys that included both male and female physicians, the rates for sexual involvement were consistently higher for males. If we assume that the actual rate of sexual mis-

Table 2. Surveys of Sexual Misconduct by Physicians

Authors; Publication Date	Physicians Surveyed	Number and Source	Sex of Respondents	Response Rate (%)	Overall Rate of Sexual Involvement with Patients (%)
Kardener et al. 1973 [92]	Fam Prac, Int Med Ob-Gyn, Psych, Surg	1,000 randomly selected from county medical society	Male	46	12.8
Perry 1976 [137]	Fam Prac, Int Med, Ped, Psych, Other	500 randomly selected from NY and CA	Female	31	0.6
Wilbers et al. 1992 [184]	Ob-Gyn, Otol	All 975 members of both Dutch specialty societies	Both	67	4
Gartrell et al. 1992 [58]	Fam Prac, Int Med, Ob-Gyn, Surg	10,000 randomly selected from AMA Physician Masterfile	Both	19	9

Lamont and Woodward 1994 [106]	Ob-Gyn	All 792 members of Society of Obstetricians and Gynaecologists of Canada	Both	78	3
Coverdale et al. 1995 [32]	Fam Prac	217 randomly selected from all New Zealand family practitioners	Both	86.2	3.8
Bayer et al. 1996 [13]	Fam Prac, Int Med, Ob-Gyn, Ophth	1,600 randomly selected from AMA Physician Masterfile	Both	52	3.4
Ovens and Permaul-Woods 1997 [132]	Emg Med	974 from commercial mailing list in Ontario, Canada	Both	61.5	6.2

Abbreviations: AMA = American Medical Association; Emg Med = Emergency Medicine; Fam Prac = Family Practice; Int Med = Internal Medicine; Ob-Gyn = Obstetrics and Gynecology; Ophth = Ophthalmology; Otol = Otolaryngology; Ped = Pediatrics; Psych = Psychiatry; Surg = Surgery conduct is greater than the lowest rates acknowledged in these surveys, then some 5 to 10 percent of male physicians have adulterated the doctor-patient relationship.

How Common Is Sexual Misconduct by Practicing Psychiatrists? Table 3 summarizes the results of three surveys of practicing psychiatrists about their sexual involvement with current or former patients. (The survey by Judith Perry listed in table 2 is not included because it does not give response rates by specialty. None of the 30 female psychiatrists in that study acknowledged sexual involvement with their patients.) Based on these three surveys, the rate of sexual misconduct by male psychiatrists is about 10 percent.

As a point of comparison, four self-report surveys of practicing psychologists carried out between 1977 and 1986 revealed that 4.8 to 12 percent of males and 0.8 to 3 percent of females had been sexually involved with current or former patients [21; 85; 139; 140].

How Common Is Sexual Misconduct by Psychiatry Residents? To my knowledge, there has been only one survey of sexual misconduct by psychiatry residents. In that study, Nanette Gartrell and her colleagues sent a self-report questionnaire to all 1,113 PGY-4 residents listed in the 1986 American Medical Association Physician Masterfile [57]. Of the 1,087 questionnaires that were delivered, 548 (50.4%) were returned, though not all respondents answered every question. Overall, 72.1 percent of the residents (85.7% of the males and 52.0% of the females) acknowledged having been sexually attracted to one or more patients. Most of these residents (78.3%) discussed their attraction with their supervisors—a discussion that was more likely if the resident had been in psychotherapy.

Five of 539 residents (0.9%) admitted to sexual involvement with patients. In two cases (a single heterosexual male and a married heterosexual male), the misconduct occurred in the PGY-4 year; in one case (a separated or divorced heterosexual female), it occurred in the PGY-1 year; in one case (a single homosexual male), it occurred during a medical student clerkship on psychiatry; and in one case (a married heterosexual male),

Table 3. Surveys of Sexual Misconduct by Practicing Psychiatrists

Authors; Publication Date	Number and Source of Potential Respondents	Response Rate (%)	Rate of Sexual Involvement for Males (%)	Rate of Sexual Involvement for Females (%)
Kardener et al. 1973 [92]	200 males randomly selected from county medical society	57	10	—
Gartrell et al. 1986 [56]	5,574 psychiatrists selected by every fifth name from AMA Physician Masterfile	26	7.1	3.1
Leggett 1994 [107]	506 Fellows of the RANZCP selected by every third name from Australian Fellows List	68	9.3	1.4

Abbreviations: AMA = American Medical Association; RANZCP = Royal Australian and New Zealand College of Psychiatrists

the timing was not specified. The rate of sexual involvement acknowledged by residents was considerably lower than that reported by practicing psychiatrists—almost certainly because the residents had less exposure to patients than their seniors had. In recent years psychiatry residency programs have given more attention to preventing sexual misconduct [63; 64; 145; 177], but it remains for future surveys to discover whether such efforts have been effective.

Is Sexual Involvement with Former Patients Sexual Misconduct? Some of the surveys listed in tables 2 and 3 asked physicians (including psychiatrists) whether they approved or disapproved of sexual involvement with patients. Although most physicians condemned such behavior with current patients, fewer believed it was inappropriate with former patients. In addition to those surveys, there have been two reports that have focused on the subject in greater detail. The first, by John Coverdale and his colleagues [31], surveyed 500 obstetrician-gynecologists, 500 ophthalmologists, 250 internists, and 250 family practitioners. The names of these physicians were randomly selected from the American Medical Association Physician Masterfile, and the sample was limited to physicians under fifty years of age. Of the 1,500 questionnaires sent out, 777 were returned, for an overall response rate of 53.7 percent. Questionnaires were completed by 257 obstetrician-gynecologists (51.4%), 259 ophthalmologists (51.8%), 127 internists (50.8%), and 134 family practitioners (53.6%). Although both male and female physicians were surveyed, the findings were not analyzed by the sex of the respondent.

The investigators asked whether certain behaviors were *usually, sometimes,* or *never appropriate* at several stages of the doctor-patient relationship, or whether the respondent had *no opinion* on the matter. Some of the results of this survey are summarized in table 4. I find them disturbing because so many physicians thought that sexual involvement—or behavior that could lead to it—was acceptable conduct with current or former patients.

The second report to focus on physicians' attitudes about sexual involvement with patients dealt exclusively with psychiatrists. This report, by Judith Herman and her colleagues [80], was part of the survey summarized in table 3 with Nanette Gartrell as the first author. As noted in that table, the investigators sent a questionnaire to 5,574 psychiatrists who were selected by taking every fifth name from the American Medical Association Physician Masterfile. Completed questionnaires were returned by 1,423 psychiatrists, for a response rate of 26 percent.

Table 4. Physicians' Approval of Certain Behaviors with Current or Former Patients

Behavior	*Physician Groups* Who Thought Behavior Was Sometimes or Usually Appropriate (%)*
During consultation	
Arranging to meet for lunch	31.7–46.3
Kissing	13.4–21.8
Sexual contact	0.0–0.8
While patient in treatment	
Meeting for lunch	47.1–56.4
Kissing	19.7–31.3
Sexual contact	3.2–12.5
After patient left treatment	
Meeting for lunch	73.9–82.8
Kissing	58.3–71.5
Sexual contact	47.0–59.1

Source: Modified with permission from John Coverdale et al., "National Survey on Physicians' Attitudes toward Social and Sexual Contact with Patients," *Southern Medical Journal* 87, no. 11 (1994): 1067–71.
*Groups consisted of 257 obstetrician-gynecologists, 259 ophthalmologists, 127 internists, and 134 family practitioners.

In the survey, sexual contact was defined as "contact which [is] intended to arouse or satisfy sexual desire in the patient, therapist, or both" [56, p. 1127]. Despite the clarity of this definition, some of the findings reported by Herman and her colleagues are presented in a contradictory way. On the one hand, the investigators note that 98 percent of the psychiatrists surveyed believed that sexual contact was always inappropriate during consultations or while the patient was in treatment. On the other hand, they note that 11 percent of the respondents believed that kissing a patient could be appropriate in some circumstances and that "less than 5% believed that fondling, sitting on a lap, disrobing, or genital contact is appropriate under any circumstances" [80, p. 165]. Although these two sets of findings seem difficult to reconcile, it is clear that the great majority of respondents disapproved of sexual contact with patients who were in treatment.

Herman and her colleagues also found that the majority of psychiatrists surveyed disapproved of sexual contact with patients who had left treatment: 64.6 percent thought that it was inappropriate, 26.9 percent thought that it could sometimes be appropriate, and 8.5 percent had no opinion on the matter. As with the physicians in other specialties surveyed by Coverdale and his colleagues, there was less censure of sexual contact with former patients than there was of such contact with current patients, but, across the board, psychiatrists were more disapproving of sexual involvement at any stage in the doctor-patient relationship than were nonpsychiatric physicians.

Even though more psychiatrists regarded sexual involvement with former patients as sexual misconduct than other physicians did, I take little comfort from the thought that a sizable number of my colleagues could find such behavior acceptable. For me, the most important thing is not that the psychiatrist and the patient are both adults, or that true love can happen at any time, or that the patient might have an acute problem that can be quickly and permanently resolved—for me, the most important thing is what it means to be a psychiatrist.

I understand that psychiatrists sometimes do things that, in the psychiatric context, are roughly equivalent to an ophthalmologist's removing a cinder from a patient's eye. Thus, a psychiatrist might do a single consultation on a surgical patient who has a postoperative delirium. In such cases, you could say that there is no professional relationship to speak of, so that if the psychiatrist subsequently met the patient they could ethically establish any type of nonprofessional relationship they wanted. The contrast between this situation and doing psychodynamic psychotherapy with a narcissistic patient for an hour a week, month after month, in which the most intimate details of the patient's life are discussed is clear. But what if the psychiatrist assessed the mood of a patient with major depression twice in two weeks while that patient's psychiatrist was on vacation, or saw a bereaved patient for four sessions to discuss the latter's ambivalent feelings about a deceased parent, or did eight sessions of cognitive-behavioral therapy with a phobic patient, or did three months of weekly supportive psychotherapy with a demoralized patient immediately after the latter's divorce? Would it be ethical for the psychiatrist to become sexually involved with any of these patients after the treatment ended? How would the psychiatrist know whether or not the former patient's participation in the sexual relationship was motivated by a lingering transference reaction? Would it make a difference if the psychiatrist did not believe in the concept of transference [53; 122]? Would a sexual relationship be appropriate with a 20-year-old former patient? With an 18-year-old one? Should it make any difference if the psychiatrist and the former patient live in a small town (where the psychiatrist might be the only one in practice) or in a large city? And what length of time would be needed to decide that the professional relationship—and therefore the patient's vulnerability to exploitation—was well and truly over? Is three months long enough? A year [7; 8]?

To translate all of the issues raised by such questions into a guide for ethical behavior would need a decision-tree of bewildering complexity (e.g., "If the former patient is 18 years of age or older but still living with his or her parents, and if the treatment occurred on a weekly basis and lasted between three and six months, then a sexual relationship could be established after an interval of 9 months, unless the former patient has moved back home after a divorce, in which case the interval must be 12 months"). And even if such an algorithm could be agreed upon by the nation's psychiatrists or their representatives in professional organizations, state laws would be—as they now are— quite different from one another in deciding what constitutes criminal behavior when psychotherapists have sexual relations with patients.

My major disagreement with an "algorithmic" approach to sexual misconduct is more fundamental than that it would be unwieldy and unworkable. In my view, the most important problem is that it would bury under a mountain of petty distinctions the question of what it means to be a psychiatrist. In the matter of treating patients, psychiatrists should be more concerned with their responsibilities than their rights. The best way for all psychiatrists to meet their responsibility to protect patients from exploitation is to hold that, once a person becomes a patient, that individual loses *forever* the potential to become certain other things—an intimate friend, a lover, a spouse, an adopted child, an employee, a business partner. There are many other people who can fill these roles in our lives, and we should turn to *them* for confiding, romantic, and commercial relationships. We expect that patients will trust us, and we must make it clear that they can. In my opinion, sexual involvement with former patients *is* sexual misconduct and I therefore support the position of the American Psychiatric Association: "Sexual activity with a current or former patient is unethical" [6, p. 5].

What to Do If the Patient Takes the Initiative. It can be very unsettling when patients communicate by dress, speech, or behavior that they want you to cross the boundary of the psychotherapeutic relationship. If it seems that the patient is sending a message indirectly, it is always possible that you have misinterpreted an innocent phenomenon. If you ignore it and wait to see if it occurs again, you can minimize the risk of such a mistake. Even if your interpretation is correct, ignoring it allows the patient to save face if he or she has misjudged you and permits you to decide whether, with this patient at this time in this type of psychotherapy, you want to pursue the matter in subsequent sessions or finesse it—assuming the message is never sent again.

The odds may be greater that something in the patient's dress, speech, or behavior is an invitation for you to leave the psychiatrist's role if it represents a change from the patient's baseline. A patient who has worn transparent blouses or unbuttoned shirts from the very first session may dress that way every day, and even though the patient is sending a message (and one that may eventually become a topic for discussion in psychotherapy), it is not necessarily an invitation for you to abandon the role of psychiatrist. When that something in the patient's dress is new, however, and you are sure that it does not reflect the beginning of a hypomanic episode or a state of intoxication, you should ask about it if the phenomenon is repeated. Your inquiry will be less awkward if it is introduced with a transition from something the patient has said (e.g., "On the subject of work, I noticed that, both last week and today, you wore a transparent blouse/unbuttoned shirt. Were you trying to send a message to a co-worker—or to someone else?"). In the discussion that follows, you may learn that the change in the patient's dress was provoked by a slighting remark from a friend and that the patient now wants to prove that he or she is attractive despite what the friend thinks. In such cases, the patient's change in dress is not intended specifically for you, and it need not lead to a discussion of what is appropriate in the psychotherapeutic relationship. When the change *is* intended specifically for you, it may not have an erotic goal (e.g., "You always seem so cool and distant. I just wanted to see if you were a human being—if you'd react.") or it may, indeed, have such a goal (e.g., "Well, I was hoping that you'd notice me as a man/woman rather than just a patient. And to tell the truth, I think you're very attractive."). In either of the latter two cases, you should review the ground rules for a psychotherapeutic relationship and decide with the patient whether he or she is committed to following them.

The same general approach can be adopted if the patient seems to be sending an indirect message through speech (e.g., calling you by your first name) or behavior (e.g., touching your arm as you open the door after the session). Here, it is possible that the patient is not inviting you to cross the boundary of the psychotherapeutic relationship but has merely spoken or acted spontaneously out of friendly, grateful, or affectionate feelings. When patients who make such gestures respect the boundaries of the relationship, they may become embarrassed or apologize for their unwarranted familiarity, and the incident is never repeated. Of course, patients who *are* indirectly inviting a different kind of relationship can also apologize (to permit a graceful retreat if rebuffed), but—all things considered—it might be better to reserve a discussion about the respective roles of psychiatrist and patient until the speech or behavior occurs a second time.

When the patient sends a direct message, through speech or action, that he or she wants to have physical contact with you or wants you to be a friend or a lover, your response should be equally direct. Spoken invitations can be introduced in a variety of ways:

- "This relationship is so lopsided—you know everything about me and I don't know anything about you. I want to get to know you—the *real* you."
- "I think you'd understand me a lot better if we spent some time together out of the office."
- "I feel so lonely. Nobody cares about me. You say you care about me, but you don't show it."

Statements such as these should prompt a review of the psychotherapeutic relationship and a discussion of why the patient's other relationships are not providing what he or she wants from you.

Although it is always important to document the significant events and themes of each session in your notes, it is especially important to record, verbatim, a patient's invitation for you to cross the psychotherapeutic boundary and how you responded to it. You should do this immediately following the session in order to make it as accurate as possible—something that may be of great help if a disappointed patient retaliates by falsely accusing you of a sexual impropriety [14; 70; 158].

Careful documentation is, if anything, even more important when the patient's invitation is enacted rather than spoken. The medicolegal situation today is little different from that in 1993, when Thomas Gutheil and Glen Gabbard cautioned:

From the viewpoint of current risk-management principles, a handshake is about the limit of social physical contact at this time. Of course, a patient who attempts a hug in the last session after 7 years of intense, intensive, and successful therapy should probably not be hurled across the room. However, most hugs from patients should be discouraged in tactful, gentle ways by words, body language, positioning, and so forth. Patients who deliberately or provocatively throw their arms around the therapist despite repeated efforts at discouragement should be stopped. An appropriate response is to step back, catch both wrists in your hands, cross the patient's wrists in front of you, so that the crossed arms form a barrier between bodies, and say firmly, "Therapy is a talking relationship; please sit down so we can discuss your not doing this any more." [71, p. 195]

It is the responsibility of the psychiatrist, not the patient, to prevent sexual involvement. When a patient takes the initiative in trying to change the nature of your relationship, you must discuss the matter with your psychotherapy supervisor and residency director before you see the patient again. These discussions will permit you to talk through an unsettling experience and get advice about what to do next. You should then note in the patient's chart that the discussions have taken place and the reasoning behind the approach you will use in upcoming sessions. If, despite your best efforts, the patient persists in speech or behavior that undermines the psychotherapeutic relationship, treatment should be terminated, with appropriate referral to another psychotherapist.

What to Do If You Want to Take the Initiative. You can—and will—have any number of unprofessional thoughts about your patients, but what you say and what you do should be entirely professional. Because the capacity of psychiatrists for self-deception and post-hoc justification is probably no different from that of anyone else, it is not surprising that some psychiatrists guilty of sexual misconduct have defended their actions as beneficial to their patients. In the survey conducted by Nanette Gartrell and her colleagues, for example, although 73 percent of the psychiatrists who had been sexually involved with patients reported that love or pleasure had been their motivation, 19 percent said that it had been "to enhance the patient's self-esteem and/or to provide a restitutive emotional experience for the patient" [56, p. 1128].

If you are lonely and want company, are troubled and want understanding, are wounded and want comfort, or are lustful and want release, you must never take advantage of a patient to obtain it. If there is no one else in your life to provide what you desire, never ask a patient to furnish it. If a patient's problems are sexual in nature, you must help resolve them as a psychiatrist, not as a surrogate. And even when you sense or know that a patient would readily comply with your wishes, you must never forget that the patient is just that—a patient.

If sexual thoughts about a patient interfere with your clinical reasoning, or if you worry that you might act on those thoughts, you must discuss your predicament with your psychotherapy supervisor and residency director. They should understand how such thoughts can develop in the context of psychotherapy [157], and they will help you decide how best to proceed. You may feel embarrassed to seek their advice, but the stakes for the patient, and for you, are very high.

The Use of First Names

There are issues other than sexual misconduct that should lead you to reflect on the boundaries of the psychotherapeutic relationship. One such issue is the use of first names. Although it is natural and appropriate to address children by their first names, I recommend that for adults you use titles (Mr., Mrs., Miss, etc.). I make this suggestion even though a survey of psychotherapists in Massachusetts revealed that most psychologists, many social workers, and some psychiatrists routinely called patients by their first names [159], and surveys of Australian and British psychiatric inpatients showed that the great majority of them wanted to be called by their first names [61; 147].

One reason I think it is better to address adult patients formally is to provide a measure of symmetry in what is a most asymmetrical relationship. Because patients will, almost without exception, address you by your title, you should address them by theirs. In so doing, you will demonstrate that you regard them as adults and, in the end, as equals.

Another reason to use titles when addressing adult patients is that none of them will be offended by it, whereas some (especially those older than you) could feel demeaned if you call them by their first names. It would be quite difficult for many patients, especially at the start of a psychotherapeutic relationship, to protest and insist that you use their titles.

A final reason for addressing adult patients formally is to remind them of the professional nature of the relationship. When some patients (e.g., dependent or histrionic ones) are called by their first names, it may be easier for them to think of you as a kind of parent, friend, or potential lover who will magically solve their problems. A similar blurring of boundaries can occur if you try to obtain a measure of symmetry in the relationship by asking patients to call you by *your* first name. What you hope to convey by doing this and what the patient actually makes of it may be very different things.

Even when adult patients ask to be called by their first names, as they sometimes do on meeting you, I still think it is wise to use titles because at that point you have no idea why they are making the request. You can respond to a patient who asks to be called by his or her first name in a straightforward manner:

Psychiatrist: Hello, Mr. Franklin. I'm Alice Henry.
Patient: Hello, Doc.
Psychiatrist: Have a seat.
Patient: Thanks.
Psychiatrist: Did you sign in with the secretary?
Patient: Yes. She was very nice.
Psychiatrist: I'm glad to hear it. Well, Mr. Franklin, I know that Dr. Gomez referred you to the clinic because he thought you might be depressed, but I'd like you to tell me yourself what's been troubling you.
Patient: Sure, Doc, but you don't have to call me Mr. Franklin —you can just call me Charlie.
Psychiatrist: I appreciate the offer, Mr. Franklin, but in a pro-

fessional relationship like this, where you're going to call me Doctor, I'd like to call you Mister. I hope that's all right.
Patient: Sure, Doc—it's just that most doctors call me Charlie.
Psychiatrist: Well, this doctor is going to call you Mr. Franklin. Okay?
Patient: Okay.

Your Dress and Grooming

As a physician, you dress not only for yourself but also for your role. Because your role is more specifically that of a resident physician, your dress is determined, to a greater or lesser degree, by the expectations of your program. Thus, for example, the wearing of a white coat may be encouraged in one residency and discouraged in another. Whatever the expectations of your program, your dress and grooming should not hamper your relationship with patients. It is one thing to wear a religious symbol; it would be quite another to wear a tongue stud.

Surveys of general medical patients have revealed that, among patients who express a preference about the dress of their physicians, most want them to look "professional" (i.e., to dress more, rather than less, formally) [36; 116; 118]. I could find only two surveys of patients' attitudes about the dress of psychiatrists: one found that 49 British urban inpatients preferred more formal attire [61]; the other found that 58 Australian rural outpatients preferred less formal attire [142]. No general conclusion can be drawn from these two small studies except perhaps that opinions can vary with locale.

The best way to make sure that your appearance does not impede the psychotherapeutic relationship is to put yourself in your patients' shoes and imagine what effect it might have on them. Because patients in different places might have somewhat different standards about what kind of dress and grooming are appropriate for physicians, your appearance should approximate local norms. If your dress and grooming differ greatly from those norms, your patients may make assumptions about you (e.g., that you lack respect for them, that you are not serious about your work) which could be quite wrong.

Your Office

Because your office, like your dress and grooming, says something about you, you may wonder how its decor affects the psychotherapeutic relationship. Should the desk be positioned between you and the patient or against the wall? Should you display pictures of family members? Although psychiatrists now seem less concerned with such questions than they were a generation or two ago [96], it is still important to think about the layout and appearance of your office from a patient's point of view.

The matter is complicated to some extent by the fact that you are a resident, which means not only that you change offices several times a year but also that the offices you occupy have already been furnished and painted to someone else's taste and budget. Despite these constraints, you can still put your personal stamp on your surroundings.

Although the arrangement of furniture in an office (e.g., how close the chairs are to one another, where the desk is placed) would seem to have a measurable effect on the comfort levels of psychotherapists and patients, such relationships have been studied only in simulated or single-session interviews, not in actual, ongoing psychotherapy [59; 151]. Even without such studies, however, you know by now how a certain type of environment affects you, and in some cases you can tell—or guess—how it affects your patients. A paranoid patient, for example, may be more comfortable if he or she has unimpeded access to the door and is seated on the opposite side of the desk from you.

In the end, because you spend much more time in your office than any of your patients do, you should arrange and decorate it to suit your needs and preferences. It will make little difference to patients whether you have diplomas, Impressionist prints, or departmental schedules on the wall, but they might be disenchanted to see that you left a pile of clothes in the corner after a night on duty.

Self-Disclosure

I use the term *self-disclosure* here to refer to things that you reveal about yourself by what you say (e.g., that you play the piano, that your parents divorced when you were nine) rather than things you reveal about yourself by how you speak (e.g., that you grew up in the South, that you are a stickler for grammar), how you dress (e.g., that you like blue, that you are a Christian), or how you decorate your office (e.g., that you are messy, that you graduated from Ohio State).

You can disclose things about yourself because a patient asks you to or because you decide to. Most patients want to know more about their psychiatrists than can be deduced from posters on the wall or photographs on the desk, but not much more. They may ask you to reveal information that is, in a sense, public (e.g., where you went to medical school, when you will finish your residency) or somewhat private (e.g., the ages of your children, whether you enjoyed your vacation), but they usually do not ask you to reveal information that is truly private (e.g., the state of your marriage, how much money you make), either because they know it is inappropriate to do so or because they have no interest in such matters.

Many psychiatrists readily reveal public and somewhat private information in response to a patient's request when they judge the disclosure to be helpful or neutral in terms of the psychotherapeutic relationship. Those same psychiatrists, however, usually refuse to reveal truly private information, not only because they believe it would erode the boundary of the psychotherapeutic relationship but also because they know it might make it harder to discover the patient's motivation for asking. One reason why a patient might ask about your most private life is that he or she has fantasies about being your friend, or sibling, or lover, and so wants to know more about you as a person rather than as a psychiatrist. Another reason might be that the patient fears that he or she will break down if the discussion continues on its current line and asks a question to change the subject. If, in the hope of making a therapeutic point or of demonstrating your commitment to a symmetrical relationship, you disclose the private information the patient has requested, you may find that *your* life, rather than that of the patient, has become the focus of the session:

> *Patient:* We're always talking about problems with my marriage—what about your marriage? Don't you ever quarrel with your husband?
>
> *Psychiatrist:* Of course I do, every once in a while.
>
> *Patient:* Well, what do you quarrel about? I bet it's the same things—the kids, money, sex. Do you want sex every time he does?

You can deflect such questions and still preserve the opportunity to discover the patient's motivation for asking:

> *Patient:* We're always talking about problems with my marriage—what about your marriage? Don't you ever quarrel with your husband?
>
> *Psychiatrist:* What difference would it make if I did or I didn't?
>
> *Patient:* Well, if you did, maybe I wouldn't feel like I was the only one who couldn't make a man happy.
>
> *Psychiatrist:* Make a man happy?
>
> *Patient:* Isn't that what you're supposed to do? My mother didn't have a life of her own because she was supposed to make my father happy. I don't want to end up like her!

In addition to disclosing information at the request of patients, you can also disclose it without being asked. Such voluntary disclosures should not be taken lightly, for there is an important difference between saying what you think or feel as a psychiatrist and saying what you think or feel as a private individual. As a psychiatrist, you must convey certain thoughts and emotions to patients in order to help them change. Thus, it is perfectly appropriate to say that you are worried to hear that a patient has decided on a dangerous course of action or that you are happy to hear that a patient has achieved a long-sought goal.

The disclosure of these feelings keeps the focus on the patient and leads naturally to a further discussion of the patient's situation (e.g., "Now that you've got the job, do you anticipate any problems?").

There are a few circumstances in which psychiatrists, *as* psychiatrists, volunteer private information because such disclosures are common in those circumstances and are made to benefit patients. If, for example, you work in a substance abuse program because you were an alcoholic and want to help other alcoholics, you might reveal your own history to patients as evidence that you can understand their problem and as proof that someone can overcome an addiction. In making this disclosure, you would almost certainly be acting like other psychotherapists in the program who had been addicts themselves.

There are also a few circumstances in which psychiatrists, *as* psychiatrists, have a duty to volunteer private information because patients, *as* patients, have a right to know it. If, for example, you believe on religious grounds that abortion is murder, that women who have abortions are sinful, and that it is your responsibility to prevent abortions, you must disclose that information to patients considering abortions. Those patients have a right to know that your advice on the subject may be based on religious rather than clinical principles, and they should be asked if, under the circumstances, they wish to be treated elsewhere. Another example of voluntary disclosure of private information that patients have a right to know is that you have a sustained feeling about the patient (e.g., love, mistrust) that has compromised your professional judgment. If this occurs, the patient must be referred to another psychotherapist.

Voluntary disclosures of private information such as those illustrated above preserve the boundaries of the psychotherapeutic relationship. There are also, however, voluntary disclosures that violate those boundaries. It is, for example, inappropriate for psychiatrists to tell patients that they are sexually attracted to them, unless that is given as the reason for terminating treatment. Although it has been argued that such disclosures (e.g., "I think you should know I'm feeling sexually aroused right now. Are you aware that you've been acting seductively?") can be therapeutically useful, I believe that they are much more likely to have the opposite effect. Many patients would think it unprofessional for a psychiatrist to reveal sexual feelings, while others would be threatened by the revelation or use it as the basis for fantasies or behaviors that distract them from their original goals in treatment. Psychiatrists who are excited by the possibility of sexual conquest, who long for sympathetic understanding, or who are greedy for power over others may make disclosures that gratify their own needs at the expense of those of their patients. Such actions exploit the psychotherapeutic relationship to take advantage of people who have made themselves vulnerable in order to be helped. In my opinion, most inappropriate self-disclosures are not made with predatory intent, but on the basis of therapeutic zeal or naïveté. Although it is always important to think twice before disclosing private information, psychiatrists should be especially reflective when their own relationships are failing, when they are ill, when their work no longer satisfies them, or when they are suffering financial difficulties [18; 180]. If you are in doubt whether or not to disclose private information or think you have done so inappropriately, you should discuss the matter with your psychotherapy supervisor.

Calls at Home

One of the things you and your patients must discuss at the start of treatment is how they can contact you in case of emergency. Depending on your personality, your current rotation, your living arrangements, among other factors, some of you will give patients your telephone or pager number; others of you will ask them to call the hospital's answering service or emergency room. And depending on your assessment of a given patient's personality and clinical state, you will set a higher or lower threshold for such contacts—a threshold that may vary over the course of treatment. Even though you and your patients agree on the indications for calling you at night or on weekends, some of them will do it less often than you think they should, while others will do it more often than you wish them to.

There are many reasons why patients might want to speak to you outside of scheduled psychotherapy sessions. It may be, for example, that they are suicidal and want to be stopped; that they feel overwhelmed and want support; that they are paralyzed by doubt and need advice; that they are angry with you and want to punish you by disrupting your life; that they are in love with you and want to hear your voice. If a patient calls repeatedly and appropriately in the midst of a crisis, you should consider scheduling the calls—something that will reassure the patient of your availability and spare you unexpected interruptions.

Whenever patients call you at home, there is a chance that they will speak to or hear your housemate, spouse, or children. Although this might lead the patient to ask for private information you would not have volunteered, you can often deal with the request in a matter-of-fact way. Thus, for example, if a patient phones you at home and asks if the person who answered was your spouse, you can simply say, "Yes" or "No, it was my sister" and direct the conversation back to the reason for the patient's call. If, in the psychotherapy session following that call, the patient wants to know the name of your spouse or sister, you can provide it (or not) and again redirect the conversation. Most patients understand the boundaries of the psychotherapeutic relationship and will be satisfied with a minimum of information. If patients request more information than you wish to disclose, you can remind them of the nature of the psychotherapeutic relationship (e.g., that it is an asymmetrical one) and again direct the conversation to the patient's situation.

Whenever a patient phones you at home and other people are present, you should take the call in a private setting, both to assure the patient that he or she has your full attention and to minimize the chance that the patient will draw erroneous conclusions about you from voices or sounds in the background. You might also reduce the chance of erroneous conclusions if the message on your telephone answering machine is reasonably dignified.

Chance Meetings

Although chance meetings between psychiatrists and patients are more likely in small towns than in large cities, you can bump into patients no matter where you live. When you encounter patients in a mall, at a movie, in a restaurant, or at a party, the situation can be awkward—both for the patients and for you. Your behavior in these circumstances is generally best guided by what the patients do. Some of them will not acknowledge you because they too want privacy, but in the next psychotherapy session they may mention that they saw you in such-and-such a place and ask who you were with. Other patients will greet you and exchange a few words. If you are alone when this occurs, there is usually no problem, but if you are with your spouse or a friend, it gets more complicated. The best thing to do when you have a companion is simply to introduce the parties by name, but not to disclose that the patient is a patient (e.g., "Frank, this is Barbara Saunders. Mrs. Saunders, this is my husband, Frank Chen."). Spouses often know the names of patients (e.g., because they have called you at home) or quickly learn that your manner of introducing patients identifies them as such. If you are with an inquisitive friend when you meet a patient and you wish to protect the patient's status, you can simply tell the friend that the patient is someone you know from the hospital. All of this is much easier, of course, if the patients decide to identify themselves as patients when you introduce them to your companion.

If you treat students or house officers at your medical school, chance meetings on campus are common but easily dealt with, for you and the patient can exchange greetings that reflect your roles in the institution, rather than your roles in psychotherapy. When you encounter such patients at parties, however, things can be quite awkward, for you and the patient will be constrained by your psychotherapeutic relationship at the same time that other partygoers may be encouraging you to hold forth or to unwind. If that occurs, you can change the subject or excuse yourself from the conversation—actions the patient may take as well. You and the patient can then discuss the encounter in the next psychotherapy session and decide how to deal with similar situations in the future. Treating colleagues—or the family members of colleagues—is a fact of life for many physicians. In such circumstances you may well be able to manage the dual role of distant colleague and psychiatrist, but you should never attempt to be the psychiatrist of a close colleague or a friend.

Accepting Gifts

Patients may offer you small gifts on holidays, after you have expressed an interest in their hobbies, when they are especially appreciative of your efforts on their behalf, and on completion of treatment. Such gifts should generally be accepted in the spirit in which they are offered, rather than made the focus of psychotherapeutic inquiry (e.g., "Perhaps you could tell me what you were thinking when you chose the candy?"). Most psychiatrists are probably much more reluctant to accept a gift certificate than, say, a box of homemade cookies, but they might accept the gift certificate if it has a personal quality. Thus, for example, if a patient offers you a gift certificate to a restaurant, he or she may say, "It's one of my favorite places. I hope you'll enjoy it, too." Patients rarely offer cash as a gift, which is fortunate because most psychiatrists would refuse it (e.g., "I appreciate the thought, but you already pay me for my services, so I'm afraid I can't accept it"). If a patient entreats you to take a cash gift after you have declined it, you can suggest that the patient give it to a worthy cause in your name.

There are, of course, situations in which a gift should be refused and the patient's reason for offering it should be explored. A patient may, for example, try to give you something session after session or press you to accept an expensive gift. Such behavior might express a vulnerability in the patient's personality (e.g., a tendency to curry favor with authority figures that later leads to self-loathing) or it might be an attempt on the patient's part to convert a professional relationship into a personal one.

4. Psychotherapy Supervision

Learning psychotherapy is like learning surgery: although you can read about it in articles and books, mastery comes with supervised experience. Because the process of acquiring experience is a long one, it is not surprising that some beginning residents embrace a "school" of psychotherapy in hopes that knowledge of its theories and techniques will confer mastery more quickly. These hopes may be encouraged by supervisors who believe that their effectiveness as psychotherapists is derived from the teachings of the school to which they belong. This is an understandable opinion, but one that may well be incorrect, for (as noted in chapter 3) there is evidence to suggest that the relationship between the psychotherapist and the patient is a more important determinant of outcome than the theories or techniques the psychotherapist employs. Although I have discussed some aspects of psychotherapeutic theory in connection with life-story reasoning and the psychotherapeutic relationship, I return to the subject of theory here in order to examine its influence on beginning residents and their supervisors.

Psychotherapeutic Theories: Positives and Negatives

Psychotherapeutic theories can help beginners by closing gaps in a patient's life story. If, for example, you are puzzled by a female patient's domineering behavior toward the men in her life despite their evident high regard for her as a daughter, a sister, a wife, and a colleague, your familiarity with a variety of psychotherapeutic theories would allow you to consider themes that could account for the paradox. One such theme, Alfred Adler's concept of "masculine protest" [1, pp. 87–88], might permit you to connect the patient's behavior with her belief that, because it is still a male-dominated world, the only way she can overcome her feelings of inferiority is to act as she thinks a man would

act—assertively. This meaningful connection would bring co-
herence to the patient's life story and thereby contribute to its
"narrative truth" (see chapter 1). Once you can tell a coherent
story, you feel more confident that you are on the right track.

Another way—albeit a dangerous one—in which psychotherapeutic theories can increase the confidence of beginners
was suggested by Jerome Frank:

> A therapist can succeed only if he has some conviction that
> what he is doing makes sense and that he is competent to do
> it. He gains this feeling first of all from his therapeutic suc-
> cesses, which, often erroneously, he regards as evidence for
> the validity of his theory. That is, a patient's improvement may
> actually have resulted from aspects of the therapeutic situa-
> tion that escape the therapist's formulations and even his no-
> tice, such as the rebirth of hope. The success rate of most psy-
> chotherapists, however, is scarcely large enough to sustain
> their self-confidence. It is a rare therapist who has not expe-
> rienced periods of discouragement and self-doubt. At such
> moments . . . adherence to a doctrine may be a major source
> of emotional support, and the most supportive, hence the
> most seductive, theories explain away the therapist's failures
> while letting him take credit for his successes. That is, suc-
> cesses are proof of the theory's validity while failures cannot
> shake it. [43, pp. 147–48]

Beginners who embrace a psychotherapeutic theory that pur-
ports to explain all emotional distress in terms of a few simple
ideas become very confident, and very limited, psychotherapists.
Such beginners know in advance why patients are suffering and
tell the same life story for all of them. When this happens, patients disappear as individuals and become mere exemplars of
the story's main theme, whether of castration anxiety, birth
trauma, the persona and the anima, or repressed sexual abuse.
Hilde Bruch warned beginners of this danger as it applies to psychoanalysis, but her point is valid for all psychotherapeutic
theories:

Learning specific theories and therapeutic techniques, psychoanalytic or otherwise, may be stimulating and give the reassurance that one has been let in on some secret knowledge; to some it may be of help in organizing observations. But the beginner needs to realize that this knowledge does not give him any help when he sits down with a patient. It does not tell you what to say to a patient or what to listen for, and it may even make you focus on something which, according to the theory, should be there and thus stand in the way of hearing what the patient is trying to say. . . .

On the surface it may not seem to matter whether one refers to Mr. X as doing or saying this or that, or whether one speaks of his having strong or weak ego functions. The telling difference is that in one image the patient is conceived of as a person who is living his own life, though inefficiently and beset with all kinds of problems; in the other, the person is conceived of as a container that houses the various "mechanisms" or "ego functions" which determine what he does. [23, p. 85]

One of the best psychotherapy supervisors I had as a resident was a very experienced psychoanalyst who shared Bruch's opinion about the place of theory in the education of beginners. Whenever I asked him whether a patient's behavior represented, say, "identification with the aggressor," he would gently turn aside the question and ask me how I understood the behavior in terms of the patient's personality, family relationships, and social circumstances. He was very interested in *exactly* what she said and did, and his interpretations and predictions were always grounded in the particulars of the case, rather than in theoretical constructs. I had no doubt that he knew psychoanalytic theory, but what he was teaching me was the product of twenty-five years of experience as a psychotherapist.

Psychotherapeutic Theories and Clinical Experience

In 1950, Fred Fiedler published three small studies examining the relative importance of psychotherapeutic theories and clinical experience in determining the relationship psychotherapists attempt to create with their patients. In the first two studies [41], he found that psychologists and psychiatrists from a variety of backgrounds (psychoanalytic, Rogerian, Adlerian, eclectic) were in general agreement about statements most characteristic of an ideal psychotherapeutic relationship (e.g., "An empathic relationship"; "Therapist sticks closely to the patient's problems"; "The patient assumes an active role") and statements least characteristic of such a relationship (e.g., "An impersonal, cold relationship"; "The therapist curries favor with the patient"; "The therapist tries to impress the patient with his skill or knowledge"). He also found that well-educated people with no training as psychotherapists ranked a series of 75 statements about the psychotherapeutic relationship in the same way that psychologists and psychiatrists did. Fiedler concluded that the participants' notion of an ideal psychotherapeutic relationship was not derived from theories but from what they regarded as good interpersonal relationships in general.

In the third study [40], Fiedler used the same 75 statements about the psychotherapeutic relationship to assess actual psychotherapy sessions. He asked three psychotherapists (one each from psychoanalytic, Rogerian, and eclectic orientations) and one lay person to listen to recorded excerpts of psychotherapy sessions conducted by 10 different psychotherapists. Among the 10 were two expert psychoanalysts, two novice psychoanalysts, two expert Rogerian therapists, two novice Rogerian therapists, one expert Adlerian therapist, and one novice Adlerian therapist. After listening to each excerpt, the judges ranked the 75 statements according to whether they were the most, or the least, characteristic of the session from which the excerpt was taken. Whereas Fiedler's earlier studies had described the qualities of an ideal psychotherapeutic relationship, this study assessed the qualities of actual relationships. His analysis of the judges' ratings led Fiedler to the following conclusions:

(1) Expert psychotherapists of any of the three schools create a relationship more closely approximating the Ideal Thera-

peutic Relationship than relationships created by non-experts.

(2) The therapeutic relationship created by experts of one school resembles more closely that created by experts of other schools than it resembles relationships created by nonexperts within the same school.

(3) The most important dimension (of those measured) which differentiates experts from nonexperts is related to the therapist's ability to understand, to communicate with, and to maintain rapport with the patient. [p. 444]

These three studies suggest that experience, more than theory, determines the type of relationship expert psychotherapists attempt to establish with their patients. If this is true, and if the relationship is crucial to the success or failure of treatment, then what you want most from your psychotherapy supervisors is not their theoretical knowledge but their clinical wisdom.

The Focus of Supervision

At various times during the course of psychotherapy supervision, your supervisor will ask you to focus on the patient, on your relationship with the patient, or on yourself [68]. When you present a new patient to a supervisor, the focus is naturally on the patient, for the supervisor's primary responsibility is to help you make an accurate diagnosis, design an appropriate plan of treatment, and further the patient's progress. When that progress is slow or erratic, your supervisor may ask you to focus on your relationship with the patient, so that rather than discussing phenomena such as the patient's symptoms or changing life circumstances, you and the supervisor discuss phenomena such as the vicissitudes of the therapeutic alliance and the possibility that the patient is having a transference reaction. Sometimes when the patient is not doing well, but more often when you become demoralized or anxious about the progress of treatment, your supervisor may ask you to focus on yourself. As

I noted in chapter 2, your supervisor should be able to help you minimize your trait-related problems as they affect your care of patients without making you a patient yourself. Thus, for example, if you become discouraged because a difficult patient has shown little improvement, your supervisor may not only reassure you that the patient's personality is the main obstacle to progress but also speculate whether you might be distressed, in part, because you tend to be self-doubting and self-critical. You might have mentioned those traits yourself when discussing a different case, or your supervisor might have noticed them as he or she has gotten to know you over time. If you think the supervisor is correct, the two of you can talk about ways in which you can emphasize the benefits of those characteristics and diminish their burdens. If you think the supervisor is wrong, you should say so, and the two of you can shift your focus back to the patient or to your relationship with the patient.

In days gone by, it was more common for psychotherapy supervisors to focus on the supervisee, even at the beginning of supervision. This practice was based on the assumption, discussed in chapter 2, that psychiatrists need psychotherapy to be competent psychotherapists. Although many supervisors who made this assumption also believed that they could not—and should not—be both a teacher and a psychotherapist for their supervisees, they also believed that self-awareness was important for psychotherapists and that it was their responsibility to help their students become more self-aware. For these supervisors, the best setting in which to demonstrate the need for self-awareness was the supervisor-supervisee relationship, for both parties in that relationship could function as participant-observers. It was, I believe, such reasoning that led to an awkward exchange between one of my supervisors and me during our first meeting. I had just given what I thought was a thorough presentation of a complicated case and I was eager for his guidance. He began not by asking me for more information about the patient, nor by asking me to expand on my diagnostic formulation, nor by asking me to propose a plan of treatment—instead, he began by asking me why I had not told him the name of a psychiatrist who had briefly treated the patient the year before. When I responded that the treatment had lasted only a few sessions, that it had not gone well, and that I was not sure whether he knew the psychiatrist, who may have been unfairly criticized, he said, "Well, Phillip, the fact that you didn't tell me the psychiatrist's name says something about what you think of me." I was so nonplussed by his statement that I could only blurt out: "Um. . . . If you want me to tell you what I think of you, I'll tell you. Do you want me to tell you what I think of you?" It was now his turn to be dumbfounded (because, I believe, no resident had ever spoken to him like that before), and he only harrumphed and directed the conversation back to the patient.

If a psychotherapy supervisor insists on discussing your personality or your personal life when there seems no reason to do so, you should ask your residency director for a different supervisor, just as you should if a supervisor repeatedly misses sessions, usually falls asleep, or makes sexual advances. Fortunately, such behaviors are rare. In every residency program there should be wise, kind, experienced psychotherapy supervisors who will help you learn a difficult craft.

Fear of Criticism: A Potential Obstacle to Supervision

Most beginning residents are eager to have psychotherapy supervision, but that eagerness is often tempered by fear of criticism. As Stanley Greben has noted:

> The greatest pleasure for talented and interested residents is the regular opportunity to discuss psychotherapy cases with an experienced clinician and teacher. In the first year of residency, residents are intimidated by the expectation that they would engage in psychotherapy with any patient. Whatever little reading they have done on the subject has given them vague ideas of how to proceed, but no degree of confidence that they can adequately fill the role of psychotherapist. They are afraid that they may not be able to say anything useful

and, even more, that they may say something wrong or dam-
aging to the patient. . . . The psychotherapy hours seem hope-
lessly complicated, and they are all too aware that as careful
a record as they make of the proceedings, in order to be able
to report fairly to their supervisor, that record will be a pallid
shadow of what has actually taken place in therapy.

Residents come to their early meetings with a new supervisor with some apprehension. Will they be chided or humil-
iated? Will they be exposed as too supportive or laissez-faire?
Will their ignorance of psychoanalysis or psychodynamic psychiatry be woefully evident? [66, pp. 307–8]

To avoid criticism and shame, residents sometimes "edit"
their reports of psychotherapy sessions [74]. This practice, while
understandable, deprives both the patient and the resident of the
supervisor's best advice. The potential for omitting or fabricat-
ing material in order to avoid criticism is greatest when written
notes are used as the basis for supervision, but it is also possible
to edit audiotapes and videotapes—if not to create an impression of having done something, at least to create an impression
of not having done something. Deception is impossible, of
course, when the supervisor observes the session through a one-
way mirror or acts as co-therapist in group psychotherapy, but
in most residency programs direct supervision is the exception,
not the rule. Direct supervision demands even more time from
busy supervisors, and residents usually do not press for it, perhaps because it is the supervisory setting in which they have the
least privacy and therefore the least chance of saving face [16].

Being supervised in any fashion is uncomfortable for residents who mistake a supervisor's observations and conjectures
for criticisms. If you have this tendency, you might want to tell
your supervisor about it so that he or she can appropriately label
remarks. Of course, there *are* hypercritical supervisors, and if
you feel that you have one, you should discuss your predicament
with your residency director. In the end, it is up to the supervisor to provide an environment conducive to learning and to de-

termine what help you need most; in the end, it is up to you to be forthright.

Other Potential Obstacles to Supervision

The Attitude That Psychotherapy Is Not for Psychiatrists

The attitude that psychotherapy is not for psychiatrists has been promoted, in part, by psychiatrists themselves. There have been three elements in the growth of this opinion. First, it became clear that certain schools of psychotherapy had failed in their claims to understand the cause of psychiatric disorders and to offer effective treatments for those conditions. Second, the increasing pace of discovery in neuroscience and related fields has given us medications that can help patients in ways that psychotherapy never could. Here, for example, I mean not only that neuroleptics are useful for "psychotic" phenomena such as hallucinations and delusions but also that selective serotonin reuptake inhibitors are useful for "neurotic" phenomena such as obsessions and panic attacks. Finally, as psychiatry has become more like other medical specialties in its use of the scientific method, some psychiatrists have adopted a narrow and mistaken view of what they, as physicians, should be doing. This view depends on the following syllogism:

> Major Premise: Physicians treat diseases.
> Minor Premise: Psychiatrists are physicians.
> Conclusion: If the patient's complaints are due not to a disease (of the brain) but to problems in living, then the treatment of those complaints is a matter not for psychiatrists, but for psychologists, social workers, nurses, and other counselors.

The fundamental problem with such reasoning is, of course, in the major premise, for physicians treat patients, not diseases. Many physicians care for patients who are troubled rather than diseased, and some of those physicians are excellent psychotherapists, within the constraints of their practice.

To the extent that academic psychiatrists—especially directors of departments and residency programs—believe that psychotherapy is a thing of the past, a second-rate treatment, to that extent they will devalue the place of psychotherapy supervision in your education. For residency programs to be accredited, they must provide a certain amount of supervision, but some faculty members in programs that seek to produce "brain doctors" may look down on residents who are interested in psychotherapy, just as some faculty members in programs that sought to produce "mind doctors" once looked down on residents who were interested in neuroscience.

Another reason for the attitude that psychotherapy is not for psychiatrists is the change in medical practice brought about by managed care. As Paul Summergrad and his colleagues noted: "The major managed-care companies, for-profit and working in the private sector, do not permit residents to treat their members. Although a master's-prepared clinician is considered 'qualified,' even a senior psychiatric resident with an outstanding record from a nationally regarded institution and with much more training is considered inadequate" [171, p. 256]. One result of such policies is that fewer cases—especially those suitable for long-term psychotherapy—are available for supervision. Another result is that graduating psychiatrists increasingly believe that psychotherapy not only can be done by psychologists, social workers, nurses, and other counselors, but that it *should* be done by them. If this view becomes more widespread, the pool of psychiatrists qualified to be psychotherapy supervisors will soon diminish. (The advent of managed care has, of course, affected residency education in areas other than psychotherapy supervision [20; 83; 187].)

Prejudice, Ignorance, or Insensitivity by the Supervisor or the Resident

The race, culture, gender, or sexual orientation of the resident or supervisor can become an obstacle to supervision if either party in the relationship is prejudiced, ignorant, or insensitive about such matters. Relatively little has been written about this topic, perhaps because it is so awkward to study. It would be reassuring to believe that people who are interested in psychiatry tend to be tolerant of others in general and that psychiatrists tend to be tolerant of one another because so many of us belong to minority groups, but such beliefs have not been validated. Indeed, it is possible that diversity among psychiatrists provides more opportunity for prejudice, ignorance, and insensitivity than would exist if we were a more homogeneous group.

The one thing that cannot be doubted in all of this is that psychiatry residents are a fairly varied lot. Their diversity is reflected in the American Psychiatric Association's 2001–2002 Resident Census, which had an 83.2 percent response rate (5,766 residents) from 493 accredited residencies and fellowships [4]. That survey revealed, for example, that male and female residents were equally common, and that 38.6 percent of residents were international medical graduates. Racial identification was not provided by 7.9 percent of the respondents, but 58.0 percent identified themselves white, 24.6 percent as Asian, 6.7 percent as Black/African American, 0.4 percent as Native Hawaiian/Other Pacific Islander, 0.3 percent as American Indian/Alaska Native, and 2.1 percent as Other. Residents of Hispanic ethnicity reported a variety of racial identifications and constituted 3.3 percent of the total. The APA census did not assess sexual orientation, but a survey of all Canadian psychiatry residents with a response rate of 58.7 percent revealed that 94.3 percent of the respondents described themselves as heterosexual, 4.1 percent as homosexual, and 1.6 percent as bisexual [25].

These American and Canadian surveys provide a context for considering how prejudice, ignorance, and insensitivity about matters of race, culture, gender, or sexual orientation might interfere with psychotherapy supervision. In one of the few papers on this general topic in the last decade, Carol Nadelson and her colleagues discussed the influence of gender and sexual orientation on the supervisory process [129]. They noted, for example, that communication may be distorted when supervisors assume that residents are heterosexual. If such an assumption is evident to homosexual residents, some of them may disguise their sexual orientation or refuse to present homosexual patients for supervision. Because Nadelson and her colleagues were interested in a resident perspective on how issues of gender and sexual orientation affect the supervisory process, one of the paper's authors, Keith Ablow, conducted an informal survey of residents in the Boston area. The survey revealed, among other things, that heterosexual residents disapproved of homosexuality in supervisors of either sex, and that homosexual residents tended to prefer homosexual supervisors.

Ronald Ruskin also addressed the ways in which prejudice, ignorance, and insensitivity might interfere with psychotherapy supervision, though his focus was on race and culture rather than on gender and sexual orientation:

> The supervisee from another culture may feel misunderstood, marginalized, responded to in an indifferent or prejudicial manner, and unable to express his or her particular perspectives. Cultural divergences may make the supervisee more vigilant and anxious about the supervisor's capacity to attend to and critically evaluate the supervisee's experience and performance. When the supervisee comes from a different country, speaks a different mother tongue, is a member of a racial or ethnic minority, and/or is of a different religion from the dominant culture supervisor, the capacity to identify with the supervisor may be made more difficult than with a colleague who shares similar or convergent cultural determinants. [149, pp. 59–60]

If you find that one of your supervisors is prejudiced, ignorant, or insensitive about you or your patients and you do not want to raise the issue with the supervisor in question, you should bring the matter to the attention of your residency director. If you are correct about the supervisor, the odds are that he or she will apologize and try to do better; if you are wrong— and acknowledge it—the supervisor's self-esteem and reputation should be restored.

It is possible, of course, that *you* may be prejudiced, ignorant, or insensitive, and that your criticisms of a supervisor have less to do with that individual's skills as a teacher or clinician than with his or her race, culture, gender, or sexual orientation. If you realize you have such a problem, you are already on the road to correcting it. Depending on what you have said or how you have acted, an apology to the supervisor may or may not be appropriate. In any event, you will have learned something important about yourself.

An Impaired Supervisor

Psychiatrists are no less vulnerable to psychiatric disorders than other people are, and some psychiatrists are better at preaching the value of treatment than they are at accepting it. If your psychotherapy supervisor becomes impaired by a medical or surgical condition, he or she will almost certainly tell you about it and schedule a break in supervision or ask your residency director to provide a substitute. If, however, the impairment is due to a psychiatric disorder that distorts the supervisor's judgment, he or she may continue treating patients and supervising residents. If your supervisor is manic, profoundly depressed, very anxious, or repeatedly intoxicated, it will be obvious—and upsetting—to you. For the sake of your patients, the supervisor's patients, the supervisor, and the integrity of the residency program, you must tell your residency director what you have observed. If the impairing disorder is more subtle in its manifestations or if the supervisor tries to conceal it by missing sessions, it may take some time until you realize that he or she may be ill. In that case you will probably find it more awkward to speak to your residency director, but you should do so nonetheless. If you try to protect an impaired supervisor, you may only make matters worse.

I was able to find only two studies on the impact of impaired supervisors on residents. The first study, conducted by Kasia Kozlowska and her colleagues in Australia [100; 101], assessed many aspects of residents' experiences with patients, teachers, and peers. In 1994, the investigators sent a self-report questionnaire to all 137 house officers in New South Wales who had completed at least one year of training and to all 95 consultants (the equivalent of board-certified psychiatrists) in New South Wales who had achieved specialist status within the previous five years. Of the 232 questionnaires distributed, 178 (76.7%) were completed and returned: 110 of them from trainees (completion rate: 80.3%) and 68 from consultants (completion rate: 71.6%).

The investigators were particularly interested in the frequency of adverse experiences for trainees and specifically inquired about 20 potentially distressing situations, including that of being supervised by a consultant whose psychiatric disorder made the work environment unpleasant. Forty-five of the respondents (25.3%) endorsed having had such a supervisor, and 28 of them wrote comments on the question. These comments included the trainee's diagnostic impression of the disorder impairing the supervisor. Although the investigators did not list all of these diagnoses, they noted that in seven cases it was alcohol abuse; in another seven, depression; in six, mania; in four, personality disorder; and in one, "psychosis." Three of the respondents said that the impaired supervisor's colleagues did not intervene in the situation.

In the second study on the impact of impaired supervisors on residents, Karine Igartua sent a self-report questionnaire to all 600 psychiatry residents enrolled in Canadian programs in the 1996–1997 academic year [90]. The questionnaire asked, among other things, whether the resident's clinical work had been supervised by an impaired psychiatrist. In order to minimize possible confusion about the term *impairment,* Igartua provided a definition proposed by the American Medical Association's Council on Mental Health: "inability to practice medicine adequately by reason of physical or mental illness, including alcoholism or drug dependence" [3, p. 684].

Two hundred and twenty-nine residents returned the questionnaire, for a response rate of 38.2 percent. Seventeen residents (7.4%) reported having worked with impaired supervisors, and six of those residents said they developed anxiety or depression as a result. The great majority of residents who worked with impaired supervisors tried to cope with the situation by doing without supervision, by sharing their feelings, and by seeking supervision from other staff members or senior residents. In addition, almost all of them (15 of 17) felt that other staff were too passive in dealing with the situation. Fourteen of the affected residents were ambivalent about reporting their supervisors, but 12 of them did so.

Igartua understood the methodological limitations of her study, but she also saw its potential implications: "The low response rate (38%) makes it difficult to draw conclusions. However, if we presuppose that none of the nonresponders had worked with impaired supervisors, the risk of working with an impaired supervisor during residency training would be 4%" [90, p. 192]. Had Kozlowska and her colleagues made the same assumption, the risk of working with an impaired supervisor during training would be about 19 percent. If the risk for residents in general is somewhere between those two figures, and if you are in a residency program of average size, the chances are that at least one of your colleagues has an impaired supervisor.

Sexual Harassment by a Supervisor

The concept of sexual harassment includes behaviors that are gender-related, unwanted, and occur in a context where one person has power over another [10, p. S6]. Such behaviors can be verbal (e.g., making a sexist joke, commenting on someone's dress or physique, making a sexual proposition) or nonverbal (e.g., using offensive body language, touching). Although there have been many surveys of sexual harassment experienced by medical students and house officers in general, none has focused on psychiatry residents and their psychotherapy supervisors. In some studies, such as those by Deborah Cook and her colleagues [29] and Steven Daugherty and his colleagues [34], psychiatry residents were included among the house officers surveyed, but the results were not analyzed by specialty. And although Kozlowska and her colleagues assessed sexual harassment in their survey of adverse experiences for psychiatry trainees [101], it is not clear to what extent the harassment was perpetrated by peers, senior psychiatrists, nurses, or other staff.

To my knowledge, only one survey specifically investigated the sexual harassment of psychiatry residents by their teachers. In that study, Melanie Carr and her colleagues sent a self-report questionnaire to all 535 residents enrolled in Canadian programs [25]. Three hundred fourteen questionnaires were returned, for a response rate of 58.7 percent. The respondents included 169 males and 145 females. Two hundred and ninety-six of them (94.3%) described themselves as heterosexual, 13 (4.1%) as homosexual, and five (1.6%) as bisexual. Eighty-two residents were in the PGY-1 year, 76 in the PGY-2 year, 68 in the PGY-3 year, and 88 in the PGY-4 year.

Although the major focus of the survey was sexual involvement of residents with their teachers (see below), the investigators also asked about sexual harassment. A teacher ("psychiatric educator") was defined as a clinical supervisor, a course instructor, an advisor, or a residency program administrator; the term *sexual harassment* was not defined. Twenty-one of the 314 respondents (6.7%) reported that they had been propositioned by a teacher. Of this group, 19 were females (13.1% of female respondents) and two were males (1.2% of male respondents). In addition, 14 female respondents (9.7%) said that they had been sexually harassed by a teacher, whereas no male respondents did.

When a teacher violates the boundaries of the student-teacher relationship, the student is often upset and uncertain what to do next. The distressing and complicated nature of this situation is illustrated in the study conducted by Deborah Cook and her colleagues of all residents in programs sponsored by McMaster University during the 1993–1994 academic year [29]. The investigators surveyed 225 residents in seven programs (anesthesia, family medicine, internal medicine, obstetrics and gynecology, pediatrics, psychiatry, and surgery) about a variety of topics, including sexual harassment. One hundred and eighty-six residents (82.7%) returned the questionnaire, with response rates ranging from 69.0 percent for family medicine to 100 percent for anesthesia and internal medicine. The rates were almost equal for male and female residents: for males, 93 of 111 (83.8%); for females, 93 of 114 (81.6%).

One hundred and eighty-four residents completed at least some of the questions regarding 14 events the investigators thought could be experienced as sexual harassment. One hundred and seventy-one of these residents (92.9%) reported experiencing one or more such events, the most common of which were sexist jokes, compliments on the resident's physique, flirtation, and body language deemed offensive. More male residents (11.0%) than female residents (6.5%) reported having been made an explicit sexual proposition, but the difference was not statistically significant. There was no relationship between the type of residency program and the frequency of any of the 14 events. The investigators did not ask the respondents to identify the type of person (e.g., supervising physician, resident, nurse, other staff member, patient, patient's relative) responsible for the event.

One hundred and fifty-four residents described their emotional responses to these events. The most common reactions were embarrassment (24.0%), anger (23.4%), frustration (20.8%), anxiety (16.2%), feeling violated (11.0%), and helplessness (7.1%). Significantly more females than males reported feelings of anger, frustration, violation, and helplessness, whereas significantly more males than females stated that the events had made no emotional impact on them.

Of the 171 residents who reported events defined as sexual harassment, 165 answered the question that dealt with whether they had told anyone about the event. Seventy-nine of these 165 (47.9%) stated they had, and 78 of them indicated whom they had told. The most common confidants were other residents (70.5% of cases), friends (65.4%), partners or family members (53.8%), and supervising physicians (23.1%).

When respondents were asked why they had not made a formal complaint about the most distressing event they had experienced, 123 provided reasons. Most often, it was because they did not consider the behavior in question to be a problem (45.5% of cases), because they thought it was too small a problem to worry about (30.9%), because they believed that making a formal complaint would not accomplish anything (25.2%), because they thought that complaining was more trouble than it was worth (18.7%), or because they feared that complaining would adversely affect their evaluations (13.8%). Seventeen of the 123 (13.8%) said they did not make a formal complaint of sexual harassment because they had dealt with the matter themselves.

The survey conducted by Cook and her colleagues illustrates not only how distressing and complicated it can be for residents to deal with sexual harassment, but also how residents (among others) can disagree about what sexual harassment is. Although Cook and her colleagues listed 14 events as examples of sexual harassment, it seems that many of the residents who experienced some of those events did not regard them as such. Thus, certain residents might have thought that a sexist joke was gauche or boorish behavior but not sexual harassment.

If you believe a teacher's conduct toward you is sexual harassment, your decision to confront the teacher or tell your residency director will probably depend on several factors. You may be less likely to protest, for example, if the behavior is a single offensive joke than if it is a repeated sexual proposition; you may be less likely to protest if you are a forgiving or passive person than if you are a censorious or assertive one; and you may be less likely to protest if you have a distant relationship with your residency director than if you have a close one.

I urge you to confide in your residency director if you have been sexually harassed by a teacher or if you are uncertain whether a teacher's behavior constitutes sexual harassment. It is much more likely that you will be hurt by the unwanted comments, propositions, or actions of someone whose behavior should merit your respect (a category of persons that includes other residents as well as teachers) than it is that you will be hurt by reporting misconduct to someone who is responsible for your welfare as a resident.

Sexual Involvement with a Supervisor

Although sexual harassment of residents by psychotherapy supervisors can be unequivocally condemned because it is unwanted and imposed, what if a resident and supervisor establish a sexual relationship by mutual consent? Do you believe that, given the power differential between students and teachers, the resident cannot be an equal partner in the relationship, or do you believe that two adults may do as they wish, even if one happens to be the pupil of the other? Questions such as these prompted three groups of investigators to survey psychiatry residents about sexual involvement with their teachers.

The first of these studies, by Nanette Gartrell and her colleagues [57], was based on a self-report questionnaire sent to all 1,113 PGY-4 residents listed in the 1986 American Medical Association Physician Masterfile. Of the 1,087 questionnaires that were delivered, 548 (50.4%) were returned, though not all respondents answered every question. Three hundred and twenty-one respondents (58.6%) were male, 225 (41.1%) were female, and two (0.4%) did not specify their sex. Relatively more female residents (57.7%) than male residents (44.4%) returned the questionnaire.

The major focus of the survey was on sexual involvement of residents with their teachers, but it also asked about sexual involvement of residents with their patients. As I noted in chapter 3, 0.9 percent of the respondents acknowledged having been sexually involved with patients. In what follows, I will summarize the findings of the survey in relation to residents' sexual involvement with teachers. The investigators defined sexual involvement ("sexual contact") as behavior "intended to arouse or satisfy sexual desire" [p. 691]. They defined a teacher ("psychiatric educator") as a clinical supervisor, a course instructor, an advisor, or a residency program administrator. (These two definitions were subsequently used by Melanie Carr and her colleagues in their survey of Canadian psychiatry residents—a survey whose findings on sexual harassment were summarized above and whose findings on sexual relationships with teachers are summarized below.)

Gartrell and her colleagues found that almost three-quarters (74.2%) of the respondents in their survey believed that sexual involvement with a current teacher was inappropriate, but even more (80.0%) believed that such involvement could be appropriate if the resident and teacher did not have an ongoing work relationship. Male and female respondents were of the same opinion in regard to these issues.

As to the question of whether they had been sexually involved with their teachers, 26 (4.9%) of 527 respondents acknowledged that they had. (See table 5.) Fourteen of these residents were female (6.3% of female respondents) and 12 were male (3.9% of male respondents). In 14 cases, the sexual contact occurred between female residents and male teachers; in nine cases, between male residents and female teachers; in two cases, between male residents and male teachers; and in one case the respondent did not specify the sex of either party. The contact was initiated more often by the teacher when the resident was female (9 of 14 cases) than when the resident was male (2 of 11 cases).

Sexual involvement of residents with teachers often occurred early in the resident's training. Of the twenty-two respondents who specified when the involvement began, seven were in the PGY-1 year, five were in the PGY-2 year, eight were in the PGY-3 year, and two were in the PGY-4 year. Only 12 respondents identified the role of the teacher at the time: in seven cases it was as a clinical supervisor; in two cases, as a course instructor; in two cases, as an administrator; and in one case, as an advisor. In 11 cases the involvement began during a work relationship; in 14 cases it did not; and in one case the respondent did not answer the question.

Respondents were asked what they thought about the involvement at the time it occurred and were permitted to give multiple answers to this question. More respondents believed the relationship was "appropriate" (16), "caring" (11), or "helpful" (3) than believed it was "inappropriate" (2), "exploitative" (2), or "harmful" (1). When asked what they thought about the involvement at the time they filled out the questionnaire, fewer residents believed it had been "appropriate" (9), "caring" (8), or "helpful" (3), and more believed it had been "inappropriate" (7), "exploitative" (7), or "harmful" (7). At the time they filled out the questionnaire, 13 respondents were no longer sexually involved with their teachers, seven were, and six did not answer the ques-

Table 5. Surveys of Sexual Involvement of Residents with Teachers

Authors; Publication Date	Number and Source of Potential Respondents	Response Rate (%)	Rate of Residents' Sexual Involvement (%)
Gartrell et al. 1988 [57]	All 1,113 PGY-4 residents in 1986 AMA Physician Masterfile	50.4	4.9
Carr et al. 1991 [25]	All 535 Canadian psychiatry residents	58.7	2.5
Kozlowska et al. 1997 [101]	All 137 house officers in New South Wales with at least one year of training; all 95 consultant psychiatrists in New South Wales certified within last five years	76.7	2.8

Abbreviations: AMA = American Medical Association

tion. Four of the respondents were currently married to the teachers with whom they had been involved.

In the second survey of sexual involvement of psychiatry residents with their teachers, Melanie Carr and her colleagues sent a self-report questionnaire to all 535 residents enrolled in Canadian programs [25]. Three hundred and fourteen questionnaires were returned, for a response rate of 58.7 percent. The respondents included 169 males and 145 females. Two hundred and ninety-six of them (94.3%) described themselves as heterosexual, 13 (4.1%) as homosexual, and five (1.6%) as bisexual. Eighty-two residents were in the PGY-1 year, 76 in the PGY-2 year, 68 in the PGY-3 year, and 88 in the PGY-4 year.

Seventy respondents (22.3%) thought that sexual involvement of residents with teachers was unethical under any circumstances; 11 (3.5%) thought it was permissible in special circumstances (a concept not defined in the paper); eight (2.5%) thought it was permissible outside of supervisory sessions; 80 (25.5%) thought it was permissible if the teacher was not a direct supervisor; and 115 (36.6%) thought it was permissible if the supervisory relationship had been terminated. The investigators did not comment on the responses of the remaining 30 residents (9.6%).

Eight respondents (2.5%) acknowledged a total of nine sexual relationships with their teachers. (See table 5.) Six of those residents were female (4.1% of female respondents) and two were male (1.2% of male respondents). One of the female residents reported having had sexual relationships with two teachers. All of the relationships were heterosexual.

At the time of the involvement, one resident was in the PGY-1 year; two in the PGY-2 year; two in the PGY-3 year; and three in the PGY-4 year. In five cases, the teacher was the resident's supervisor, and in two of these cases the teacher was also the resident's psychotherapy supervisor. In the remaining three cases the teacher's role was not specified.

In five of the nine relationships, the sexual involvement was mutually initiated; in four of the relationships, it was initiated by the teacher. Information about the duration of the involvement was reported for seven relationships: in two, it was limited to a single contact; in four, it lasted three months; and in one, it lasted three years and resulted in marriage.

At the time the respondents filled out the questionnaire, four were no longer in contact with the teachers; one had a work relationship but no sexual involvement; two had sexual involvement but no work relationship; and two had both sexual involvement and a work relationship. Looking back on the sexual involvement with their teachers, six of the respondents had positive feelings, one had mixed feelings (i.e., that the relationship had been caring but harmful and inappropriate), and one had neutral feelings. Five of the respondents had not told anyone of their involvement; three had told friends. None of the eight respondents who had been sexually involved with their teachers expressed any regrets.

The third survey of sexual involvement of psychiatry residents with their teachers was conducted in 1994 by Kasia Kozlowska and her colleagues in Australia [100; 101]. Some of the results of that survey, which assessed many aspects of a resident's experience with patients, teachers, and peers, are summarized above in the section on impaired supervisors.

Kozlowska and her colleagues sent a self-report questionnaire to all 137 house officers in New South Wales who had completed at least one year of training, and to all 95 consultants (the equivalent of board-certified psychiatrists) in New South Wales who had achieved specialist status within the previous five years. Of the 232 questionnaires sent out, 178 (76.7%) were completed and returned: 110 of them from trainees (response rate: 80.3%) and 68 from consultants (response rate: 71.6%).

Of the 178 respondents, five (2.8%) acknowledged a sexual relationship with a senior colleague. (See table 5.) Other than noting that all of the respondents involved were female, that one of the relationships ended in marriage, and that another relationship contributed to the respondent's decision to leave psychiatry, the investigators provided no other information, perhaps because their survey was so wide-ranging that they had to sacrifice depth of inquiry for breadth.

These three surveys suggest that it is relatively uncommon for psychiatry residents to become sexually involved with their supervisors. The question remains, however, whether such relationships ought to be seen as acceptable or unacceptable. Kozlowska and her colleagues did not attempt to answer the question, but the other groups of investigators did. For both of them, the sexual involvement of residents and supervisors was a matter not only of student-teacher relationships but also of professional responsibility. Gartrell and her colleagues took an unambiguous position on the question: "Sexual contact between a psychiatric educator and resident is unethical as long as the educator has authority over the resident. We recognize that such authority may be of long duration, continuing as long as the educator is in a position to advance or obstruct the student's professional career" [57, p. 694]. Carr and her colleagues were less direct in their disapproval, but their conclusion was clear: "Departmental policies concerning sexual contact are necessary to ensure the protection of residents during the vulnerable training period. Above all, professional integrity and ethical accountability are not only learned through the intellectual examination of issues but incorporated by example. The supervisory relationship in resident education deserves careful scrutiny in this regard" [25, p. 219].

The American Psychiatric Association's publication *The Principles of Medical Ethics with Annotations Especially Applicable to Psychiatry* does not prohibit sexual relationships between residents and supervisors, but it does warn against them:

> Sexual involvement between a faculty member or supervisor and a trainee or student, in those situations in which an abuse of power can occur, often takes advantage of inequalities in the working relationship and may be unethical because—
> a. Any treatment of a patient being supervised may be deleteriously affected.
> b. It may damage the trust relationship between teacher and student.
> c. Teachers are important professional role models for their trainees and affect their trainees' future professional behavior. [6, p. 9]

Given the vulnerability of some residents to exploitation and the tendency of some psychiatrists to take advantage of those (whether patients or students) for whom they have responsibility, such warnings are appropriate. Still, residents are adults, and adults are presumed to be competent to choose their own relationships. This position was vigorously advanced by Christopher Ryan, who grounded his argument in the principle of autonomy, but even Ryan found two reasons to condemn the sexual involvement of psychiatry residents with current supervisors:

The first concerns the psychiatrist's role as a supervisor. The psychiatrist-supervisor has a primary role in shaping the trainee's development and reporting to the training body regarding the trainee's progress. A supervisor's ability to complete these tasks will be impaired if they are, or have been, their trainee's lover. . . . A supervisor involved in a sexual relationship with a trainee will not be able to give dispassionate and effective feedback either to the training body or to the trainee. . . .

There is also the possibility that a sexual relationship may result in harm to patients under the care of the trainee that the psychiatrist is supervising. The supervisor may be less able to identify mistakes made by the trainee. In addition, the trainee may be more likely to withhold information concerning adverse events in their therapeutic contacts so as to appear to their supervisor in a better light. [150, pp. 387–88]

Psychotherapy supervision is a delicate process for both student and teacher: the former must trust and take risks; the latter, encourage and criticize. All of this is hard enough without sexual involvement. If you and your psychotherapy supervisor find one another so attractive that you cannot postpone a romantic relationship until you are no longer working together, I suggest that both of you discuss the matter with your residency director and department director. This discussion will either facilitate the relationship (e.g., by assigning you another supervisor, by changing your rotation schedule) or make it clear that such relationships are frowned upon or proscribed. If a secret romantic relationship goes badly, with negative consequences for you, your supervisor, or your patients, the residency director and department director may be less sympathetic than if they had known about the relationship beforehand.

Epilogue

Becoming a psychotherapist takes practice, supervision, and patience. You must learn to balance engagement and detachment. Theory and technique are important, but they are less important than common sense and character.

Although much depends on you, patients who do not apply themselves will not improve. Psychotherapy is more like rehabilitation medicine than it is like surgery.

Becoming a psychotherapist, like becoming a physician, means learning to deal with failure. And even when a course of psychotherapy has a happy ending, there may be times when your confidence falters and you cannot sleep because you fear you have made a mistake. I have been a psychotherapist for more than thirty years, but I still ask my colleagues for advice.

Psychotherapy is the most personal of treatments, for both you and your patients. As such, it is a risky business. Listen before you speak. Think before you act. It is precisely because psychotherapy is so personal, so risky, that it can provide such great satisfaction. I wish you well.

References

1. Adler, Alfred. *Problems of Neurosis.* Edited by Philippe Mairet. With a prefatory essay by F. G. Crookshank. New York: Cosmopolitan Book Corporation, 1930.

2. Alden, Lynn. "Short-Term Structured Treatment for Avoidant Personality Disorder." *Journal of Consulting and Clinical Psychology* 57 (1989): 756–64.

3. American Medical Association, Council on Mental Health. "The Sick Physician: Impairment by Psychiatric Disorders, Including Alcoholism and Drug Dependence." *Journal of the American Medical Association* 223 (1973): 684–87.

4. American Psychiatric Association. *Census of Psychiatry Residents: 2001–2002.* Arlington, VA: American Psychiatric Association, 2003.

5. American Psychiatric Association. *Diagnostic and Statistical Manual of Mental Disorders.* 4th ed. Washington, DC: American Psychiatric Association, 1994.

6. American Psychiatric Association. *The Principles of Medical Ethics: With Annotations Especially Applicable to Psychiatry.* Washington, DC: American Psychiatric Association, 2001.

7. Appelbaum, Paul S., and Jorgenson, Linda. "Psychotherapist-Patient Sexual Contact after Termination of Treatment: An Analysis and a Proposal." *American Journal of Psychiatry* 148 (1991): 1466–73.

8. Appelbaum, Paul S.; Jorgenson, Linda M.; and Sutherland, Pamela K. "Sexual Relationships between Physicians and Patients." *Archives of Internal Medicine* 154 (1994): 2561–65.

9. Bachrach, Henry M. "Empathy: We Know What We Mean, But What Do We Measure?" *Archives of General Psychiatry* 33 (1976): 35–38.

10. Baldwin, DeWitt C., Jr., and Daugherty, Steven R. "Distinguishing Sexual Harassment from Discrimination: A Factor-Analytic Study of Residents' Reports." *Academic Medicine,* October Supplement (2001).

11. Barber, Jacques P.; Connolly, Mary Beth; Crits-Christoph,

Paul; Gladis, Lynn; and Siqueland, Lynne. "Alliance Predicts Patients' Outcome Beyond In-Treatment Change in Symptoms." *Journal of Consulting and Clinical Psychology* 68 (2000): 1027–32.

12. Bateman, Anthony W., and Fonagy, Peter. "Effectiveness of Psychotherapeutic Treatment of Personality Disorder." *British Journal of Psychiatry* 177 (2000): 138–43.

13. Bayer, Timothy; Coverdale, John; and Chiang, Elizabeth. "A National Survey of Physicians' Behaviors regarding Sexual Contact with Patients." *Southern Medical Journal* 89 (1996): 977–82.

14. Berland, David I., and Guskin, Karen. "Patient Allegations of Sexual Abuse against Psychiatric Hospital Staff." *General Hospital Psychiatry* 16 (1994): 335–39.

15. Bernstein, David P.; Kasapis, Chrysoula; Bergman, Andrea; Weld, Ellen; Mitropoulou, Vivian; Horvath, Thomas; Klar, Howard M.; Silverman, Jeremy; and Siever, Larry J. "Assessing Axis II Disorders by Informant Interview." *Journal of Personality Disorders* 11 (1997): 158–67.

16. Betcher, R. William, and Zinberg, Norman E. "Supervision and Privacy in Psychotherapy Training." *American Journal of Psychiatry* 145 (1988): 796–803.

17. Beutler, Larry E.; Machado, Paulo P. P.; and Neufeldt, Susan Allstetter. "Therapist Variables." In *Handbook of Psychotherapy and Behavior Change*, 4th ed., edited by Allen E. Bergin and Sol L. Garfield, 229–69. New York: John Wiley and Sons, 1994.

18. Blatt, Sidney J. "Commentary: The Therapeutic Process and Professional Boundary Guidelines." *Journal of the American Academy of Psychiatry and the Law* 29 (2001): 290–93.

19. Bordin, Edward S. "The Generalizability of the Psychoanalytic Concept of the Working Alliance." *Psychotherapy: Theory, Research and Practice* 16 (1979): 252–60.

20. Borus, Jonathan F. "Economics and Psychiatric Education: The Irresistible Force Meets the Moveable Object." *Harvard Review of Psychiatry* 2 (1994): 15–21.

21. Bouhoutsos, Jacqueline; Holroyd, Jean; Lerman, Hannah; Forer, Bertram R.; and Greenberg, Mimi. "Sexual Intimacy between Psychotherapists and Patients." *Professional Psychology: Research and Practice* 14 (1983): 185–96.

22. Breuer, Josef. "Fräulein Anna O." In *The Standard Edition of the Complete Psychological Works of Sigmund Freud*. Translated and

edited by James Strachey, 2:21–47. 1955. 24 vols. London: Hogarth Press and the Institute of Psycho-Analysis, 1953–74.

23. Bruch, Hilde. *Learning Psychotherapy: Rationale and Ground Rules.* Cambridge, MA: Harvard University Press, 1974.

24. Carney, Francis L. "Outpatient Treatment of the Aggressive Offender." *American Journal of Psychotherapy* 31 (1977): 265–74.

25. Carr, Melanie L.; Robinson, G. Erlick; Stewart, Donna E.; and Kussin, Dennis. "A Survey of Canadian Psychiatric Residents regarding Resident-Educator Sexual Contact." *American Journal of Psychiatry* 148 (1991): 216–20.

26. Chessick, Richard D. "Psychoanalytic Peregrinations I: Transference and Transference Neurosis Revisited." *Journal of the American Academy of Psychoanalysis* 30 (2002): 83–97.

27. Childress, Robert, and Gillis, John S. "A Study of Pretherapy Role Induction as an Influence Process." *Journal of Clinical Psychology* 33 (1977): 540–44.

28. Cleckley, Hervey. *The Mask of Sanity: An Attempt to Clarify Some Issues about the So-Called Psychopathic Personality.* 4th ed. St. Louis: C. V. Mosby, 1964.

29. Cook, Deborah J.; Liutkus, Joanne F.; Risdon, Catherine L.; Griffith, Lauren E.; Guyatt, Gordon H.; and Walter, Stephen D. "Residents' Experiences of Abuse, Discrimination and Sexual Harassment during Residency Training." *Canadian Medical Association Journal* 154 (1996): 1657–65.

30. Costa, Paul T., Jr., and McCrae, Robert R. *Revised NEO Personality Inventory (NEO PI-R) and NEO Five-Factor Inventory (NEO-FFI): Professional Manual.* Odessa, FL: Psychological Assessment Resources, 1992.

31. Coverdale, John; Bayer, Timothy; Chiang, Elizabeth; Thornby, John; and Bangs, Mark. "National Survey on Physicians' Attitudes toward Social and Sexual Contact with Patients." *Southern Medical Journal* 87 (1994): 1067–71.

32. Coverdale, John H.; Thomson, Alex N.; and White, Gillian E. "Social and Sexual Contact between General Practitioners and Patients in New Zealand: Attitudes and Prevalence." *British Journal of General Practice* 45 (1995): 245–47.

33. Daly, Karen A. "Attitudes of U.S. Psychiatry Residencies about Personal Psychotherapy for Psychiatry Residents." *Academic Psychiatry* 22 (1998): 223–28.

34. Daugherty, Steven R.; Baldwin, DeWitt C., Jr.; and Rowley, Beverley D. "Learning, Satisfaction, and Mistreatment during Medical Internship: A National Survey of Working Conditions." *Journal of the American Medical Association* 279 (1998): 1194–99.

35. de Figueiredo, John M., and Frank, Jerome D. "Subjective Incompetence, the Clinical Hallmark of Demoralization." *Comprehensive Psychiatry* 23 (1982): 353–63.

36. Dunn, Jocelyn J.; Lee, Thomas H.; Percelay, Jack M.; Fitz, J. Gregory; and Goldman, Lee. "Patient and House Officer Attitudes on Physician Attire and Etiquette." *Journal of the American Medical Association* 257 (1987): 65–68.

37. Edelstein, Ludwig. "The Hippocratic Oath: Text, Translation and Interpretation." *Bulletin of the History of Medicine,* Supplement 1 (1943).

38. Eysenck, H. J. "Personality and Drug Effects." In *Experiments with Drugs: Studies in the Relation between Personality, Learning Theory and Drug Action,* edited by H. J. Eysenck, 1–24. Oxford: Pergamon Press, 1963.

39. Fenton, Lisa R.; Cecero, John J.; Nich, Charla; Frankforter, Tami L.; and Carroll, Kathleen M. "Perspective Is Everything: The Predictive Validity of Six Working Alliance Instruments." *Journal of Psychotherapy Practice and Research* 10 (2001): 262–68.

40. Fiedler, Fred E. "A Comparison of Therapeutic Relationships in Psychoanalytic, Nondirective and Adlerian Therapy." *Journal of Consulting Psychology* 14 (1950): 436–45.

41. Fiedler, Fred E. "The Concept of an Ideal Therapeutic Relationship." *Journal of Consulting Psychology* 14 (1950): 239–45.

42. Frances, Allen. "Categorical and Dimensional Systems of Personality Diagnosis: A Comparison." *Comprehensive Psychiatry* 23 (1982): 516–27.

43. Frank, Jerome D. "Psychotherapists Need Theories." *International Journal of Psychiatry* 9 (1970–1971): 146–49.

44. Frank, Jerome D., and Frank, Julia B. *Persuasion and Healing: A Comparative Study of Psychotherapy.* 3d ed. Baltimore: Johns Hopkins University Press, 1991.

45. Freud, Sigmund. "The Future Prospects of Psycho-Analytic Therapy." In *The Standard Edition of the Complete Psychological Works of Sigmund Freud.* Translated and edited by James Strachey, 11:139–51. 1964. 24 vols. London: Hogarth Press and the Institute of Psycho-Analysis, 1953–74.

46. Freud, Sigmund. "The Interpretation of Dreams." In *Standard Edition*, 4. 1953. *See* 45.

47. Freud, Sigmund. "On Beginning the Treatment (Further Recommendations on the Technique of Psycho-Analysis I)." In *Standard Edition*, 12:121–44. 1958. *See* 45.

48. Freud, Sigmund. "On the History of the Psycho-Analytic Movement." In *Standard Edition*, 14:7–66. 1957. *See* 45.

49. Freud, Sigmund. "The Psychotherapy of Hysteria." In *Standard Edition*, 2:253–305. 1955. *See* 45.

50. Freud, Sigmund. "Recommendations to Physicians Practising Psycho-Analysis." In *Standard Edition*, 12:109–20. 1958. *See* 45.

51. Gabbard, Glen O. "Commentary: Boundaries, Culture, and Psychotherapy." *Journal of the American Academy of Psychiatry and the Law* 29 (2001): 284–86.

52. Gabbard, Glen O. "A Contemporary Psychoanalytic Model of Countertransference." *Journal of Clinical Psychology/In Session* 57 (2001): 983–91.

53. Gabbard, Glen O. "Post-Termination Sexual Boundary Violations." *Psychiatric Clinics of North America* 25 (2002): 593–603.

54. Gabbard, Glen O. "Psychotherapy of Personality Disorders." *Journal of Psychotherapy Practice and Research* 9 (2000): 1–6.

55. Garfield, Sol L., and Bergin, Allen E. "Personal Therapy, Outcome and Some Therapist Variables." *Psychotherapy: Theory, Research and Practice* 8 (1971): 251–53.

56. Gartrell, Nanette; Herman, Judith; Olarte, Silvia; Feldstein, Michael; and Localio, Russell. "Psychiatrist-Patient Sexual Contact: Results of a National Survey, I: Prevalence." *American Journal of Psychiatry* 143 (1986): 1126–31.

57. Gartrell, Nanette; Herman, Judith; Olarte, Silvia; Localio, Russell; and Feldstein, Michael. "Psychiatric Residents' Sexual Contact with Educators and Patients: Results of a National Survey." *American Journal of Psychiatry* 145 (1988): 690–94.

58. Gartrell, Nanette K.; Milliken, Nancy; Goodson, William H., III; Thiemann, Sue; and Lo, Bernard. "Physician-Patient Sexual Contact: Prevalence and Problems." *Western Journal of Medicine* 157 (1992): 139–43.

59. Gass, Carlton S. "Therapeutic Influence as a Function of Therapist Attire and the Seating Arrangement in an Initial Interview." *Journal of Clinical Psychology* 40 (1984): 52–57.

60. Gaston, Louise. "The Concept of the Alliance and Its Role in

Psychotherapy: Theoretical and Empirical Considerations." *Psychotherapy* 27 (1990): 143–53.

61. Gledhill, Julia A.; Warner, James P.; and King, Michael. "Psychiatrists and Their Patients: Views on Forms of Dress and Address." *British Journal of Psychiatry* 171 (1997): 228–32.

62. Goethe, Johann Wolfgang von. *Wilhelm Meister's Apprenticeship.* Translated and edited by Eric A. Blackall in cooperation with Victor Lange. Princeton, NJ: Princeton University Press, 1994.

63. Gorton, Gregg E., and Samuel, Steven E. "A National Survey of Training Directors about Education for Prevention of Psychiatrist-Patient Sexual Exploitation." *Academic Psychiatry* 20 (1996): 92–98.

64. Gorton, Gregg E.; Samuel, Steven E.; and Zebrowski, Sandra M. "A Pilot Course for Residents on Sexual Feelings and Boundary Maintenance in Treatment." *Academic Psychiatry* 20 (1996): 43–55.

65. Greben, Stanley E. "On Being Therapeutic." *Canadian Psychiatric Association Journal* 22 (1977): 371–80.

66. Greben, Stanley E. "Interpersonal Aspects of the Supervision of Individual Psychotherapy." *American Journal of Psychotherapy* 45 (1991): 306–16.

67. Greenspan, Marie, and Kulish, Nancy Mann. "Factors in Premature Termination in Long-Term Psychotherapy." *Psychotherapy* 22 (1985): 75–82.

68. Group for the Advancement of Psychiatry, Committee on Medical Education. *Trends and Issues in Psychiatry Residency Programs.* Report no. 31. Topeka, KS: Group for the Advancement of Psychiatry, 1955.

69. Gunderson, John G. *Borderline Personality Disorder: A Clinical Guide.* Washington, DC: American Psychiatric Publishing, 2001.

70. Gutheil, Thomas G. "Borderline Personality Disorder, Boundary Violations, and Patient-Therapist Sex: Medicolegal Pitfalls." *American Journal of Psychiatry* 146 (1989): 597–602.

71. Gutheil, Thomas G., and Gabbard, Glen O. "The Concept of Boundaries in Clinical Practice: Theoretical and Risk-Management Dimensions." *American Journal of Psychiatry* 150 (1993): 188–96.

72. Gutheil, Thomas G., and Gabbard, Glen O. "Misuses and Misunderstandings of Boundary Theory in Clinical and Regulatory Settings." *American Journal of Psychiatry* 155 (1998): 409–14.

73. Gutheil, Thomas G., and Simon, Robert I. "Non-Sexual

Boundary Crossings and Boundary Violations: The Ethical Dimension." *Psychiatric Clinics of North America* 25 (2002): 585–92.

74. Hantoot, Mark S. "Lying in Psychotherapy Supervision: Why Residents Say One Thing and Do Another." *Academic Psychiatry* 24 (2000): 179–87.

75. Heider, Fritz, and Simmel, Marianne. "An Experimental Study of Apparent Behavior." *American Journal of Psychology* 57 (1944): 243–59.

76. Heimann, Paula. "On Counter-Transference." *International Journal of Psycho-Analysis* 31 (1950): 81–84.

77. Heine, Ralph W., ed. *The Student Physician as Psychotherapist.* Chicago: University of Chicago Press, 1962.

78. Henry, William P., and Strupp, Hans H. "The Therapeutic Alliance as Interpersonal Process." In *The Working Alliance: Theory, Research, and Practice,* edited by Adam O. Horvath and Leslie S. Greenberg, 51–84. New York: John Wiley and Sons, 1994.

79. Henry, William P.; Strupp, Hans H.; Schacht, Thomas E.; and Gaston, Louise. "Psychodynamic Approaches." In *Handbook of Psychotherapy and Behavior Change,* 4th ed., edited by Allen E. Bergin and Sol L. Garfield, 467–508. New York: John Wiley and Sons, 1994.

80. Herman, Judith Lewis; Gartrell, Nanette; Olarte, Silvia; Feldstein, Michael; and Localio, Russell. "Psychiatrist-Patient Sexual Contact: Results of a National Survey, II: Psychiatrists' Attitudes." *American Journal of Psychiatry* 144 (1987): 164–69.

81. Hill, A. B. "Extraversion and Variety-Seeking in a Monotonous Task." *British Journal of Psychology* 66 (1975): 9–13.

82. Hoehn-Saric, Rudolf; Frank, Jerome D.; Imber, Stanley D.; Nash, Earl H.; Stone, Anthony R.; and Battle, Carolyn C. "Systematic Preparation of Patients for Psychotherapy—I. Effects on Therapy Behavior and Outcome." *Journal of Psychiatric Research* 2 (1964): 267–81.

83. Hoge, Michael A.; Jacobs, Selby C.; and Belitsky, Richard. "Psychiatric Residency Training, Managed Care, and Contemporary Clinical Practice." *Psychiatric Services* 51 (2000): 1001–5.

84. Hollender, Marc H. "The Case of Anna O: A Reformulation." *American Journal of Psychiatry* 137 (1980): 797–800.

85. Holroyd, Jean Corey, and Brodsky, Annette M. "Psychologists' Attitudes and Practices Regarding Erotic and Nonerotic Physical Contact with Patients." *American Psychologist* 32 (1977): 843–49.

86. Horowitz, Mardi J. "Psychotherapy for Histrionic Personal-

ity Disorder." *Journal of Psychotherapy Practice and Research* 6 (1997): 93–107.

87. Horvath, Adam O. "Research on the Alliance." In *The Working Alliance: Theory, Research, and Practice,* edited by Adam O. Horvath and Leslie S. Greenberg, 259–86. New York: John Wiley and Sons, 1994.

88. Horvath, Adam O. "The Therapeutic Relationship: From Transference to Alliance." *Journal of Clinical Psychology/In Session* 56 (2000): 163–73.

89. Horvath, Adam O., and Symonds, B. Dianne. "Relation between Working Alliance and Outcome in Psychotherapy: A Meta-Analysis." *Journal of Counseling Psychology* 38 (1991): 139–49.

90. Igartua, Karine J. "The Impact of Impaired Supervisors on Residents." *Academic Psychiatry* 24 (2000): 188–94.

91. Jaspers, Karl. *General Psychopathology.* Translated by J. Hoenig and Marian W. Hamilton. With a new foreword by Paul R. McHugh. 2 vols. Baltimore: Johns Hopkins University Press, 1997.

92. Kardener, Sheldon H.; Fuller, Marielle; and Mensh, Ivan N. "A Survey of Physicians' Attitudes and Practices regarding Erotic and Nonerotic Contact with Patients." *American Journal of Psychiatry* 130 (1973): 1077–81.

93. Katz, Martin M.; Lorr, Maurice; and Rubinstein, Eli A. "Remainer Patient Attributes and Their Relation to Subsequent Improvement in Psychotherapy." *Journal of Consulting Psychology* 22 (1958): 411–13.

94. Kernberg, Otto F. *Borderline Conditions and Pathological Narcissism.* New York: Jason Aronson, 1975.

95. Kernberg, Otto. "Notes on Countertransference." *Journal of the American Psychoanalytic Association* 13 (1965): 38–56.

96. Kiernan, Kevin W.; Wise, Thomas, N.; and Mann, Lee S. "The Physical Layout of Psychiatric Offices: A Survey." *Psychiatric Journal of the University of Ottawa* 14 (1989): 453–55.

97. Kissane, David W.; Bloch, Sidney; Onghena, Patrick; McKenzie, Dean P.; Snyder, Ray D.; and Dowe, David L. "The Melbourne Family Grief Study, II: Psychosocial Morbidity and Grief in Bereaved Families." *American Journal of Psychiatry* 153 (1996): 659–66.

98. Kohut, Heinz. "The Two Analyses of Mr. Z." *International Journal of Psycho-Analysis* 60 (1979): 3–27.

99. Korb, Margaret P.; Gorrell, Jeffrey; and Van De Riet, Vernon.

Gestalt Therapy: Practice and Theory. 2d ed. New York: Pergamon Press, 1989.

100. Kozlowska, Kasia; Nunn, Kenneth; and Cousens, Pennelope. "Training in Psychiatry: An Examination of Trainee Perceptions. Part 1." *Australian and New Zealand Journal of Psychiatry* 31 (1997): 628–40.

101. Kozlowska, Kasia; Nunn, Kenneth; and Cousens, Pennelope. "Adverse Experiences in Psychiatric Training. Part 2." *Australian and New Zealand Journal of Psychiatry* 31 (1997): 641–52.

102. Kroll, Jerome. "Boundary Violations: A Culture-Bound Syndrome." *Journal of the American Academy of Psychiatry and the Law* 29 (2001): 274–83.

103. Kroll, Jerome. *The Challenge of the Borderline Patient: Competency in Diagnosis and Treatment.* New York: W. W. Norton, 1988.

104. Krupnick, Janice L.; Sotsky, Stuart M.; Simmens, Sam; Moyer, Janet; Elkin, Irene; Watkins, John; and Pilkonis, Paul A. "The Role of the Therapeutic Alliance in Psychotherapy and Psychotherapy Outcome: Findings in the National Institute of Mental Health Treatment of Depression Collaborative Research Program." *Journal of Consulting and Clinical Psychology* 64 (1996): 532–39.

105. Kuhn, Thomas S. *The Copernican Revolution: Planetary Astronomy in the Development of Western Thought.* Cambridge, MA: Harvard University Press, 1957.

106. Lamont, John A., and Woodward, Christel. "Patient-Physician Sexual Involvement: A Canadian Survey of Obstetrician-Gynecologists." *Canadian Medical Association Journal* 150 (1994): 1433–39.

107. Leggett, Andrew. "A Survey of Australian Psychiatrists' Attitudes and Practices Regarding Physical Contact with Patients." *Australian and New Zealand Journal of Psychiatry* 28 (1994): 488–97.

108. Liberman, Bernard L.; Frank, Jerome D.; Hoehn-Saric, Rudolf; Stone, Anthony R.; Imber, Stanley D.; and Pande, Shashi K. "Patterns of Change in Treated Psychoneurotic Patients: A Five-Year Follow-Up Investigation of the Systematic Preparation of Patients for Psychotherapy." *Journal of Consulting and Clinical Psychology* 38 (1972): 36–41.

109. Livesley, W. John. "Commentary on Reconceptualizing Personality Disorder Categories Using Trait Dimensions." *Journal of Personality* 69 (2001): 277–86.

110. Luborsky, Lester. "Helping Alliances in Psychotherapy." In

Successful Psychotherapy: Proceedings of the Ninth Annual Symposium, November 19–21, 1975, Texas Research Institute of Mental Sciences, edited by James L. Claghorn, 92–116. New York: Brunner/Mazel, 1976.

111. McCrae, Robert R., and Costa, Paul T., Jr. "Personality Trait Structure as a Human Universal." *American Psychologist* 52 (1997): 509–16.

112. McCrae, Robert R., and Costa, Paul T., Jr. "Validation of the Five-Factor Model of Personality across Instruments and Observers." *Journal of Personality and Social Psychology* 52 (1987): 81–90.

113. McCrae, Robert R.; Stone, Stephanie V.; Fagan, Peter J.; and Costa, Paul T., Jr. "Identifying Causes of Disagreement between Self-Reports and Spouse Ratings of Personality." *Journal of Personality* 66 (1998): 285–313.

114. McHugh, Paul R., and Slavney, Phillip R. *The Perspectives of Psychiatry.* 2d ed. Baltimore: Johns Hopkins University Press, 1998.

115. McKendree-Smith, Nancy L.; Floyd, Mark; and Scogin, Forrest R. "Self-Administered Treatments for Depression: A Review." *Journal of Clinical Psychology* 59 (2003): 275–88.

116. McKinstry, Brian, and Wang, Ji-Xiang. "Putting on the Style: What Patients Think of the Way Their Doctor Dresses." *British Journal of General Practice* 41 (1991): 275–78.

117. McNair, Douglas M.; Lorr, Maurice; and Callahan, Daniel M. "Patient and Therapist Influences on Quitting Psychotherapy." *Journal of Consulting Psychology* 27 (1963): 10–17.

118. McNaughton-Filion, Louise; Chen, John S. C.; and Norton, Peter G. "The Physician's Appearance." *Family Medicine* 23 (1991): 208–11.

119. Macaskill, Norman, and Macaskill, Ann. "Psychotherapists-In-Training Evaluate Their Personal Therapy: Results of a UK Study." *British Journal of Psychotherapy* 9 (1992): 133–38.

120. Macran, Susan, and Shapiro, David A. "The Role of Personal Therapy for Therapists: A Review." *British Journal of Medical Psychology* 71 (1998): 13–25.

121. Mains, Jennifer A., and Scogin, Forrest R. "The Effectiveness of Self-Administered Treatments: A Practice-Friendly Review of the Research." *Journal of Clinical Psychology/In Session* 59 (2003): 237–46.

122. Malmquist, Carl P., and Notman, Malkah T. "Psychiatrist-

Patient Boundary Issues following Treatment Termination." *American Journal of Psychiatry* 158 (2001): 1010–18.

123. Marmor, Judd. "Orality in the Hysterical Personality." *Journal of the American Psychoanalytic Association* 1 (1953): 656–71.

124. Marziali, E. "Three Viewpoints on the Therapeutic Alliance: Similarities, Differences, and Associations with Psychotherapy Outcome." *Journal of Nervous and Mental Disease* 172 (1984): 417–23.

125. Millon, Theodore, with Roger D. Davis and contributing associates Carrie M. Millon, Andrew Wenger, Maria H. Van Zuilen, Marketa Fuchs, and Renée B. Millon. *Disorders of Personality: DSM-IV and Beyond.* 2d ed. New York: John Wiley and Sons, 1996.

126. Mitchell, Kevin M.; Bozarth, Jerold D.; and Krauft, Conrad C. "A Reappraisal of the Therapeutic Effectiveness of Accurate Empathy, Nonpossessive Warmth, and Genuineness." In *Effective Psychotherapy: A Handbook of Research,* edited and with commentaries by Alan S. Gurman and Andrew M. Razin, 482–502. Oxford: Pergamon Press, 1977.

127. Moeller, F. Gerard; Dougherty, Donald M.; Lane, Scott D.; Steinberg, Joel L.; and Cherek, Don R. "Antisocial Personality Disorder and Alcohol-Induced Aggression." *Alcoholism: Clinical and Experimental Research* 22 (1998): 1898–1902.

128. Morey, Leslie C.; Gunderson, John; Quigley, Brian D.; and Lyons, Michael. "Dimensions and Categories: The 'Big Five' Factors and the *DSM* Personality Disorders." *Assessment* 7 (2000): 203–16.

129. Nadelson, Carol C.; Belitsky, Catherine; Seeman, Mary V.; and Ablow, Keith. "Gender Issues in Supervision." In *Clinical Perspectives on Psychotherapy Supervision,* edited by Stanley E. Greben and Ronald Ruskin, 41–51. Washington, DC: American Psychiatric Press, 1994.

130. Newman, Michelle G.; Erickson, Thane; Przeworski, Amy; and Dzus, Ellen. "Self-Help and Minimal-Contact Therapies for Anxiety Disorders: Is Human Contact Necessary for Therapeutic Efficacy?" *Journal of Clinical Psychology* 59 (2003): 251–74.

131. Norcross, John C.; Strausser-Kirtland, Dianne; and Missar, C. David. "The Processes and Outcomes of Psychotherapists' Personal Treatment Experiences." *Psychotherapy* 25 (1988): 36–43.

132. Ovens, Howard J., and Permaul-Woods, Joanne A. "Emergency Physicians and Sexual Involvement with Patients: An Ontario Survey." *Canadian Medical Association Journal* 157 (1997): 663–69.

133. Parkes, Colin Murray. "The First Year of Bereavement: A

Longitudinal Study of the Reaction of London Widows to the Death of Their Husbands." *Psychiatry* 33 (1970): 444–67.

134. Peebles, Mary Jo. "Personal Therapy and Ability to Display Empathy, Warmth and Genuineness in Psychotherapy." *Psychotherapy: Theory, Research and Practice* 17 (1980): 258–62.

135. Perls, Fritz. *The Gestalt Approach and Eye Witness to Therapy.* Palo Alto, CA: Science and Behavior Books, 1973.

136. Perry, J. Christopher; Banon, Elisabeth; and Ianni, Floriana. "Effectiveness of Psychotherapy for Personality Disorders." *American Journal of Psychiatry* 156 (1999): 1312–21.

137. Perry, Judith Adams. "Physicians' Erotic and Nonerotic Physical Involvement with Patients." *American Journal of Psychiatry* 133 (1976): 838–40.

138. Pfohl, Bruce; Blum, Nancee; and Zimmerman, Mark. *Structured Interview for DSM-IV Personality (SIDP-IV).* Washington, DC: American Psychiatric Press, 1997.

139. Pope, Kenneth S.; Keith-Spiegel, Patricia; and Tabachnick, Barbara G. "Sexual Attraction to Clients: The Human Therapist and the (Sometimes) Inhuman Training System." *American Psychologist* 41 (1986): 147–58.

140. Pope, Kenneth S.; Levenson, Hanna; and Schover, Leslie R. "Sexual Intimacy in Psychology Training: Results and Implications of a National Survey." *American Psychologist* 34 (1979): 682–89.

141. Quality Assurance Project. "Treatment Outlines for Paranoid, Schizotypal and Schizoid Personality Disorders." *Australian and New Zealand Journal of Psychiatry* 24 (1990): 339–50.

142. Rajagopalan, Mani; Santilli, Mario; Powell, David; Murphy, Megan; O'Brien, Marice; and Murphy, John. "Mental Health Professionals' Attire." *Australian and New Zealand Journal of Psychiatry* 32 (1998): 880–83.

143. Reich, Wilhelm. *Character Analysis.* 3d ed., enlarged. Translated by Vincent R. Carfagno. New York: Simon and Schuster, 1972.

144. Roazen, Paul. "The Problem of Silence: Training Analyses." *International Forum of Psychoanalysis* 11 (2002): 73–77.

145. Roman, Brenda, and Kay, Jerald. "Residency Education on the Prevention of Physician-Patient Sexual Misconduct." *Academic Psychiatry* 21 (1997): 26–34.

146. Rosenbaum, Max, and Muroff, Melvin, eds. *Anna O.: Fourteen Contemporary Reinterpretations.* New York: Free Press, 1984.

147. Rosenman, S. J., and Goldney, R. D. "Naming of Patients

by Therapists." *Australian and New Zealand Journal of Psychiatry* 25 (1991): 129–31.

148. Rounsaville, Bruce J.; Chevron, Eve S.; Prusoff, Brigitte A.; Elkin, Irene; Imber, Stanley; Sotsky, Stuart; and Watkins, John. "The Relation between Specific and General Dimensions of the Psychotherapy Process in Interpersonal Psychotherapy of Depression." *Journal of Consulting and Clinical Psychology* 55 (1987): 379–84.

149. Ruskin, Ronald. "Issues in Psychotherapy Supervision when Participants Are from Different Cultures." In *Clinical Perspectives on Psychotherapy Supervision,* edited by Stanley E. Greben and Ronald Ruskin, 53–72. Washington, DC: American Psychiatric Press, 1994.

150. Ryan, Christopher James. "Sex, Lies and Training Programs: The Ethics of Consensual Sexual Relationships between Psychiatrists and Trainee Psychiatrists." *Australian and New Zealand Journal of Psychiatry* 32 (1998): 387–91.

151. Ryan, William P. "Therapist's Office Is a Treatment Variable." *Psychological Reports* 45 (1979): 671–75.

152. Salzman, Leon. "Psychotherapy of the Obsessional." *American Journal of Psychotherapy* 33 (1979): 32–40.

153. Sandler, J.; Dare, C.; and Holder, A. "Basic Psychoanalytic Concepts: III. Transference." *British Journal of Psychiatry* 116 (1970): 667–72.

154. Sandler, J.; Dare, C.; and Holder, A. "Basic Psychoanalytic Concepts: IV. Counter-Transference." *British Journal of Psychiatry* 117 (1970): 83–88.

155. Sanislow, Charles A., and McGlashan, Thomas H. "Treatment Outcome of Personality Disorders." *Canadian Journal of Psychiatry* 43 (1998): 237–50.

156. Schafer, Roy. *Retelling a Life: Narration and Dialogue in Psychoanalysis.* New York: Basic Books, 1992.

157. Schwartz, Richard S., and Olds, Jacqueline. "A Phenomenology of Closeness and Its Application to Sexual Boundary Violations: A Framework for Therapists in Training." *American Journal of Psychotherapy* 56 (2002): 480–93.

158. Sederer, Lloyd I., and Libby, Mayree. "False Allegations of Sexual Misconduct: Clinical and Institutional Considerations." *Psychiatric Services* 46 (1995): 160–63.

159. Senger, Harry L. "First Name or Last? Addressing the Patient in Psychotherapy." *Comprehensive Psychiatry* 25 (1984): 38–43.

160. Shapiro, D. A. "The Effects of Therapeutic Conditions: Pos-

itive Results Revisited." *British Journal of Medical Psychology* 49 (1976): 315–23.

161. Shapiro, David. *Neurotic Styles.* New York: Basic Books, 1965.

162. Sherwood, Michael. *The Logic of Explanation in Psycho-analysis.* New York: Academic Press, 1969.

163. Simon, Robert I. "Commentary: Treatment Boundaries—Flexible Guidelines, not Rigid Standards." *Journal of the American Academy of Psychiatry and the Law* 29 (2001): 287–89.

164. Simon, Robert I. "Sexual Exploitation of Patients: How It Begins Before It Happens." *Psychiatric Annals* 19 (1989): 104–12.

165. Simon, Robert I. "Therapist-Patient Sex: From Boundary Violations to Sexual Misconduct." *Psychiatric Clinics of North America* 22 (1999): 31–47.

166. Slavney, Phillip R. *Perspectives on "Hysteria."* Baltimore: Johns Hopkins University Press, 1990.

167. Slavney, Phillip R., and McHugh, Paul R. "Life-Stories and Meaningful Connections: Reflections on a Clinical Method in Psychiatry and Medicine." *Perspectives in Biology and Medicine* 27 (1984): 279–88.

168. Sloane, R. Bruce; Cristol, Allan H.; Pepernik, Max C.; and Staples, Fred R. "Role Preparation and Expectation of Improvement in Psychotherapy." *Journal of Nervous and Mental Disease* 150 (1970): 18–26.

169. Spence, Donald P. *Narrative Truth and Historical Truth: Meaning and Interpretation in Psychoanalysis.* New York: W. W. Norton, 1982.

170. Strupp, Hans H. "The Performance of Psychiatrists and Psychologists in a Therapeutic Interview." *Journal of Clinical Psychology* 14 (1958): 219–26.

171. Summergrad, Paul; Herman, John B.; Weilburg, Jeffrey B.; and Jellinek, Michael S. "Wagons Ho: Forward on the Managed Care Trail." *General Hospital Psychiatry* 17 (1995): 251–59.

172. Tickle, Jennifer J.; Heatherton, Todd F.; and Wittenberg, Lauren G. "Can Personality Change?" In *Handbook of Personality Disorders: Theory, Research, and Treatment,* edited by W. John Livesley, 242–58. New York: Guilford Press, 2001.

173. Truax, Charles B., and Carkhuff, Robert R. *Toward Effective Counseling and Psychotherapy: Training and Practice.* Chicago: Aldine, 1967.

174. Truax, Charles B.; Wargo, Donald G.; Frank, Jerome D.; Imber, Stanley D.; Battle, Carolyn C.; Hoehn-Saric, Rudolf; Nash, Earl H.; and Stone, Anthony R. "Therapist Empathy, Genuineness, and Warmth and Patient Therapeutic Outcome." *Journal of Consulting Psychology* 30 (1966): 395–401.

175. Uhlenhuth, E. H., and Duncan, David B. "Subjective Change with Medical Student Therapists: I. Course of Relief in Psychoneurotic Outpatients." *Archives of General Psychiatry* 18 (1968): 428–38.

176. Uhlenhuth, E. H., and Duncan, David B. "Subjective Change with Medical Student Therapists: II. Some Determinants of Change in Psychoneurotic Outpatients." *Archives of General Psychiatry* 18 (1968): 532–40.

177. Vamos, Marina. "The Concept of Appropriate Professional Boundaries in Psychiatric Practice: A Pilot Training Course." *Australian and New Zealand Journal of Psychiatry* 35 (2001): 613–18.

178. Voglmaier, Martina M.; Seidman, Larry J.; Niznikiewicz, Margaret A.; Dickey, Chandlee C.; Shenton, Martha E.; and McCarley, Robert W. "Verbal and Nonverbal Neuropsychological Test Performance in Subjects with Schizotypal Personality Disorder." *American Journal of Psychiatry* 157 (2000): 787–93.

179. Voglmaier, Martina M.; Seidman, Larry J.; Salisbury, Dean; and McCarley, Robert W. "Neuropsychological Dysfunction in Schizotypal Personality Disorder: A Profile Analysis." *Biological Psychiatry* 41 (1997): 530–40.

180. Weiner, Myron F. "Personal Openness with Patients: Help or Hindrance." *Texas Medicine* 76 (1980): 60–62.

181. Weintraub, Daniel; Dixon, Lisa; Kohlhepp, Elizabeth; and Woolery, Janet. "Residents in Personal Psychotherapy: A Longitudinal and Cross-Sectional Perspective." *Academic Psychiatry* 23 (1999): 14–19.

182. Weissman, Sidney. "American Psychiatry in the 21st Century: The Discipline, Its Practice, and Its Work Force." *Bulletin of the Menninger Clinic* 58 (1994): 502–18.

183. Widiger, Thomas A. "Categorical versus Dimensional Classification: Implications from and for Research." *Journal of Personality Disorders* 6 (1992): 287–300.

184. Wilbers, D.; Veenstra, G.; van de Wiel, H. B. M.; and Weijmar Schultz, W. C. M. "Sexual Contact in the Doctor-Patient Relationship in the Netherlands." *British Medical Journal* 304 (1992): 1531–34.

185. Williams, Chris, and Whitfield, Graeme. "Written and

Computer-Based Self-Help Treatments for Depression." *British Medical Bulletin* 57 (2001): 133–44.

186. Wolberg, Lewis R. *The Technique of Psychotherapy.* 4th ed. 2 vols. Orlando, FL: Grune and Stratton, 1988.

187. Yager, Joel; Docherty, John P.; and Tischler, Gary L. "Preparing Psychiatric Residents for Managed Care: Values, Proficiencies, Curriculum, and Implications for Psychotherapy Training." *Journal of Psychotherapy Practice and Research* 6 (1997): 108–22.

188. Yeung, Albert S.; Lyons, Michael J.; Waternaux, Christine M.; Faraone, Stephen V.; and Tsuang, Ming T. "The Relationship between DSM-III Personality Disorders and the Five-Factor Model of Personality." *Comprehensive Psychiatry* 34 (1993): 227–34.

189. Zimmerman, Mark; Pfohl, Bruce; Stangl, Dalene; and Corenthal, Caryn. "Assessment of DSM-III Personality Disorders: The Importance of Interviewing an Informant." *Journal of Clinical Psychiatry* 47 (1986): 261–63.

190. Zur, Ofer, and Lazarus, Arnold A. "Six Arguments against Dual Relationships and Their Rebuttals." In *Dual Relationships and Psychotherapy,* edited by Arnold A. Lazarus and Ofer Zur, 3–24. New York: Springer, 2002.

Index

Psychotherapy (*cont.*)
psychotherapeutic theory in,
62, 68, 75–76, 107–11, 132; self-
administered, 58–60; and therapeutic alliance, 67–70. *See also*
Psychotherapeutic relationship;
Psychotherapists; Traits
Psychotherapy supervision: effect
of impaired supervisor on, 119–
21; effect of prejudiced supervisor or supervisee on, 116–19;
fear of criticism in, 113–15;
focus of, 40, 56, 111–13; and
psychotherapeutic theory, 107–
11; sexual harassment during,
121–24; sexual relationships
during, 124–31; and view that
psychotherapy should not be
done by psychiatrists, 115–16

Reich, Wilhelm, 8
Role induction, 45, 68–70, 74–75
Rosenbaum, Max, 9
Ruskin, Ronald, 118
Ryan, Christopher, 130–31

Salzman, Leon, 49
Sandler, Joseph, 72
Schizoid personality. *See* Personality
Schizotypal personality. *See* Personality
Scogin, Forrest, 59–60
Self-disclosure by psychotherapist,
100–103, 104, 105
Sexual misconduct: encouraged by
patient, 92–95; with former patients, 88–92; justified by per-
petrator of, 83, 95–96; by
nonpsychiatric physicians,
82–86, 88, 89; by practicing
psychiatrists, 86, 88–90; by
practicing psychologists, 81–82,
86; by psychiatry residents,

86–88; and "slippery slope,"
79–80, 102–3; and temptation
to engage in, 95–96; unethical
nature of, 91–92, 96. *See also*
Psychotherapists
Shapiro, David: on histrionic
personality, 41; on paranoid
personality, 26–28
Shapiro, David A., 55–56
Sherwood, Michael, 15–18
Simmel, Marianne, 2–4
Simon, Robert, 79–81
Spence, Donald, 13–14
Splitting, 37–39
Structured Interview for DSM-IV
Personality (SIDP-IV), 23–24
Sullivan, Harry Stack, 9
Summergrad, Paul, 116
Supervision. *See* Psychotherapy
supervision

Therapeutic alliance. *See* Psychotherapeutic relationship
Traits: aggressiveness, 35–36; assessed, 20–24; deceitfulness,
29–30, 34–35; defined, 20;
doubting, 49–50; emotional lability, 42–43; emotional restriction, 31; fear of being criticized,
45, 113–15; feelings of entitlement, 44–45; feelings of superiority, 43–44; impressionistic
thinking, 41–42; interaction
with situations, 19, 20, 24–25,
56, 79; inventory of, 20–22;
passivity, 46–47; preoccupation
with details, 48–49; reluctance
to take risks, 45–46; reluctance
to disagree, 47–48; secretiveness, 29–30; self-injurious behavior, 39–40; self-referential
thinking, 31–32; social detachment, 30–31; suspiciousness,
26–29; use of vague language,

Phillip R. Slavney, M.D., is the Eugene Meyer III Professor of Psychiatry and Medicine at the Johns Hopkins University School of Medicine. He was Director of Residency Education in the Department of Psychiatry and Behavioral Sciences at the Oregon Health and Science University from 1974 to 1976 and was Director of Residency Education in the Department of Psychiatry and Behavioral Sciences at the Johns Hopkins University School of Medicine from 1977 to 1993. Dr. Slavney has been a psychotherapy supervisor for more than thirty years, has published articles on psychotherapy for beginners, and is co-author with Paul R. McHugh of *The Perspectives of Psychiatry*, now in its second edition.

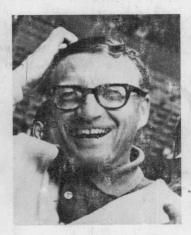

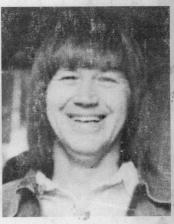

JOHN OWEN considers himself a professional writer and an amateur eater. In his profession, he is sports editor of The Seattle Post-Intelligencer. In his avocation, he produces The Intermediate Eater food column in conjunction with his wife, Alice, and with the reluctant cooperation of two test-taster offspring.

RAY COLLINS is probably the Northwest's most popular newspaper cartoonist, and a regular illustrator for The Intermediate Eater food series. He has been staff artist and cartoonist for The Seattle Post-Intelligencer for 25 years and is married to a beautiful chemical engineer, the mother of three teenagers.

INTERMEDIATE EATER

"No kitchen should be without a copy of Intermediate Eater, because I drew the pictures."

— *Ray Collins*

"John Owen certainly has an interesting way with food . . . all over my nice, clean kitchen."

— *Alice Owen*

"The ingredients in this book do not necessarily reflect the editorial policy of The Seattle Post-Intelligencer, where they first appeared."

— *The Editors*

1

Preface

The title Intermediate Eater, for the series which appears weekly in the Northwest magazine of the Sunday Seattle Post-Intelligencer, was chosen advisedly. I am not a gourmet cook. I am not even handy around the house, although I have determined that by lying on my back in the bathroom for 3½ hours I can dislodge two bolts and replace a toilet seat. If I were in the third grade at Enatai Elementary, the teacher would send me home with a note saying that my small muscles have not yet developed.

But I do have two things going for me, as the author of a cook book. I am (A) cheap and (B) usually hungry. So this book may help you avoid starvation at minimal expense. And it could even exert a considerable impact upon your life . . . or your digestion . . . if you also happen to be coconuts for garlic, oysters, clams or chili peppers.

— John Owen

WARNING—The author may have inadvertently included recipes for inconsequential and possibly healthful food, like vegetables, salads and desserts. No separate chapters have been devoted to these obviously suspect foods but they are indexed at the rear of the book.

2

INTERMEDIATE EATER

By JOHN OWEN

Illustrations by Ray Collins.

A collection of recipes which first appeared in Northwest Magazine
of The Seattle Post-Intelligencer

CONTENTS

3

Breakfasts

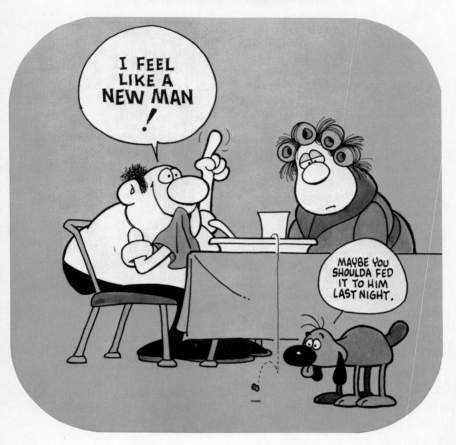

DON'T JUST sit there in a stupor each morning, with your elbow in the butter saucer. True, the symbolism and allegory in the current installment of Blondie may be a bit heavy at that hour. But you could at least pick up the cereal box and try to improve your mind.

On second thought, forget it. You'll learn that you've been stuffing yourself with sodium ascorbate for the past 11 years, and the thought may prompt the bottom of your stomach to fall out.

You've probably also been belting yourself with glycerol monosterate. Can you even guess what happens when you mix that with niacinamide and stearic acid? I know, I know. How is the average innocent dupe to suspect that something called Captain Soggy would contain pyridoxine? Expecially at 7:45 a.m., when your defenses are dulled.

Oh, well, it's your own fault. The civilized diner wouldn't touch cold cereal with a vaulting pole. The repast I chose one recent morning didn't come in a cardboard box. But if it did, the list of ingredients would read something like this:

"Contains gin, lamb kidneys, curry powder, chopped green onion and assorted nummies. Note: the minimum daily requirement for gin has not been established. But we're working on it."

Obviously, the dish is Curried Kidneys, and if you're game you might assemble two or three veal kidneys (or four to six lamb kidneys), two tablespoons of chopped green onion, two teaspoons of curry powder, one ounce of gin, 1/4 cup butter, a cup of chicken stock and some flour, to serve two.

Trim the kidneys, remove membranes (sorry about that, Gladys) and cut into bite-sized pieces. Heat the butter in a skillet, cook the onion briefly, add the curry powder and cook-stir five minutes.

Roll the kidneys in flour, toss into the skillet and cook, turning frequently, until the kidneys begin to lose color. Pour in the chicken stock, some freshly ground pepper, a few flicks of salt, to taste, and the gin.

Simmer about 10 minutes and serve in a cereal bowl with pink giraffes on the side, if you're so inclined. Or you can dump it on top of some toast or English muffins. Or you can dump it in the garbage, if you dislike kidneys, and start all over with one of the recipes on the opposite page.

Old-China Omelet

One onion
1/8 tea. crushed red pepper
1 Cup diced ham
6 eggs
One green pepper
Soy sauce
1/8 tea. salt

Slice the onion. Remove white pith and seeds from halved green pepper and cut in strips.

Saute the onion, green pepper and diced ham in frying pan with two teaspoons of oil. Sprinkle in the salt and crushed red pepper. Reduce heat to low, pour in six beaten eggs and cover pan.

When the eggs are set top with one or two tablespoons of soy sauce and serve immediately, in wedges, on warmed plates.

Belgian Waffles

5 eggs
2-1/2 cups flour
1 tea vanilla
1 cup milk
5 T. melted butter
1/4 cup powdered sugar
pinch salt

Seaparate the eggs. (After you crack them, dumb head!) Mix the egg yolks with the butter, flour, sugar, salt, vanilla and milk.

Beat the egg whites until firm and gradually stir in the batter until thoroughly mixed.

Cook in slightly buttered waffle iron and serve with syrup or, better yet, top with powdered sugar, strawberries, whipped cream, and diet until Friday. Or forget the diet and construct:

S.O.S. Rarebit

Cook and stir one pound ground beef, 1/2 cup chopped onion and one minced garlic clove in a frying pan until meat is no longer pink.

Glunk in one can of cheese soup and one-third cup milk, a few drops of tabasco, 1/4 cup catsup, salt, pepper. Stir until smooth and hot, serve over toast and sprinkle with paprika.

He was a University of Washington quarterback, a great kid, had a terrific attitude, and just one failing.

He fumbled a lot.

He was cursed with an affliction known variously as Numb Thumbs or Frozen Fingers. In the lexicon of the late departed Seattle Pilots baseball team, he had Bad Hands. The Bad Hands condition reached epidemic proportions among the Seattle Pilots.

A lot of aspiring cooks operate under the same handicap. Chances are they aren't involved in any major culinary disasters. I mean, they probably won't fall in the minestrone or dice an index finger into the tossed salad.

But there comes a disturbing moment of truth when the recipe reads:

"When lightly browned on the bottom, slip spatula underneath, deftly fold omelet in half, and serve on warm platter."

"Deft" is an unfortunate word to use around somebody with Bad Hands. Because somewhere between the sizzle and the fold he is going to rip a hole in his omelet, the culinary equivalent of a kick in the stomach. As an artistic creation, a torn omelet is Whistler's Mother, with two noses.

That's one reason the following omelet recipe is a winner. No deftness required.

Bad Hands Omelet

One medium-large zucchini will feed two. Wash it and then chop, unpeeled, into quarter-inch squares. Toss into some boiling water for three minutes, then drain in a collander, and dry with a paper towel.

Soak two tablespoons fine bread crumbs in two tablespoons of cold milk while you are lightly beating four eggs in a bowl, and pre-heating your oven broiler. Toss into another bowl the zucchini, the soaked bread crumbs, two tablespoons parmesan cheese, one-half teaspoon of grated lemon peel and one-quarter teaspoon of salt. Mix, add the beaten eggs and mix again, lightly.

Melt two tablespoons butter in a handleless skillet. When it begins to sizzle lightly, glunk in the zucchini-egg mixture.

When lightly browned on the bottom, DO NOT deftly fold it in half.

Instead, sprinkle a couple more tablespoons parmesan on top and shove the pan into the oven, three inches from the heat, for a minute, and serve.

And don't feel distraught if you drop the hot skillet halfway between the stove and the table.

You have messed up a great lunch. But some people just have Bad Hands.

8

Eye-Opener Eggs
(Serves Two)

Boil six eggs . . . yesterday.

Melt two tablespoons butter in saucepan, add one teaspoon minced onion and one peeled garlic clove. Cook briefly, remove garlic, and blend in a mixture of two tablespoons flour, ½ teaspoon of salt and 1½ teaspoons curry powder.

Oh yeah, five minutes ago you were supposed to dissolve two chicken bouillon cubes in 1¼ cups of hot water. Gradually add this to the curry mixture, stirring until thick and smooth. Slice the eggs, dump them into the pan, add ½ teaspoon of lemon juice and serve on toast.

Ham and Egg Pie

pie crust
1/2 lb. jack cheese
3 eggs
nutmeg
3 green onions
1/2 cup diced ham
1-1/2 cups half and half
salt, pepper

Make up enough of your favorite pie crust or roll out enough of the ready-made variety for one bottom crust. Line a pie plate, prick with a fork and cook five minutes in a 450 oven. You can do this much the night before when the red part of your eyes are still white.

The next morning preheat the oven again to 450. Chop the green onions, dice the cheese into small cubes and beat the eggs.

Cook the onion bits slowly in a tablespoon of butter, then dump them over the bottom of the partly cooked pie crust. Spread cheese cubes and ham over the top.

Mix together the beaten eggs, the half and half, salt, pepper and nutmeg and mix thoroughly. Pour this mess over the cheese cubes, filling the crust.

Toss it into the oven for 15 minutes, reduce heat to 350 and cook about another 15 minutes. Remove from oven, let it sit there on the counter a couple of minutes to think things over, then serve up in pie-sized wedges, maybe with some tomato juice and tabasco.

Breakfast Sandwich

1 T. oil
2 eggs beaten
1/4 cup minced ham
1/2 tea. salt
1 chopped onion
2 T. chopped green pepper
dash cayenne
1/2 cup grated jack cheese

Heat the oil in a skillet and toss in the onion, green pepper and the ham. When the onions are soft but not yet brown, pour in the beaten eggs, the salt, cayenne and cheese.

Scramble lightly and serve between pieces of lightly toasted, thin-sliced sandwich bread. The above ingredients are sufficient for two generous sandwiches.

Italian Sunrise
(To serve four)

8 slices bacon
3 T. butter
3 beaten eggs
6 T. olive oil
6 T. grated parmesan cheese
1 lb. cooked spaghetti

Cut the bacon in julienne and cook until almost crisp. Pour off the bacon grease. Add the olive oil and butter and saute the bacon a couple of minutes more.

Remove the pan from heat, stir in the grated cheese and the beaten eggs, pour immediately over the hot, drained spaghetti, toss and serve, with salt and grated pepper to taste.

Fried Potatoes Curry

Peel a clove of garlic and toss it into a frying pan with four tablespoons of butter and saute until the garlic starts to turn brown.

Remove the garlic and add four boiled, peeled and diced potatoes. Toss in three minced green onions, a teaspoon of minced lemon peel (the yellow part only), a teaspoon of chopped parsley, a generous sprinkling of nutmeg, salt and pepper.

Fry, turning occasionally, until crisp and brown. Stir in one-half teaspoon of curry powder, cook a minute longer, and serve.

Appetizers and Sandwiches

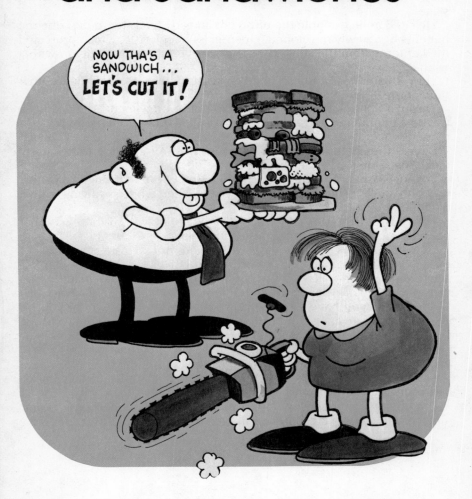

It was the opinion of no less a literary authority than Ernest Hemingway that the art of the advertising copywriter never progressed past its earliest stages.

He cited as an example the efforts of an early huckster to describe the benefits of a newly developed, green-glass beer bottle, which protected the contents from the sun's rays. The copywriter finally came up with a winner.

"Buy Bloater Beer in the new green bottle," he wrote. "Eliminates that skunk taste."

Through continuing scientific research, the brewers of America have waged a continuing and successful war against the skunk taste. But as a consequence, all beer tastes the same.

I guess there is nothing unusual about this. All gasoline tastes pretty much the same too.

But advertising campaigns have led me to believe that since I pass this way only once, I should be drinking Gusto Beer, while skydiving from a dirigible.

Yet it tastes like every other beer I've ever had, within these national boundaries, and my life continues to slip away.

The alternative is to drink wine, which does not all taste alike. In fact I make wine, in my cellar. I would recommend that all wine lovers whip off a few jugs in the cellar. There is something about homemade wine. Cheap. That's what there is about homemade wine.

And unless you have sampled homemade wine, how would you be able to appreciate an estate-bottled quart of California Cabernat Sauvignon, which doesn't turn your lips purple at the first sip? How are you going to recognize "good" unless you've encountered "awful?" Have another glass of homemade strawberry wine!

And just so it doesn't eat out the bottom of your stomach, you'd better belt yourself with the hors d'oeuvres.

The chef recommends a pound of Pike Place spoon cheese, some tuna-stuffed eggs and a chafing dish beef dip.

Saute a pound and [...] and a minced and smashed c[...] meat has lost its redness. Po[...]

    12 oz. tomato sauc[...]
    1/2 tea. salt
    1/2 cup catsup
    1 tea. Worcestersh[...]
    1 tea. oregano
    couple dashes Tab[...]
    1 tea. sugar

Simmer 15 minutes, [...] cream cheese. Heat briefly just until it begins to steam, then glunk it into the chafing dish and surround with large-sized corn chips, for dipping. That's why it's called chafing dish dip.

Tuna Stuffed Eggs

This is called tuna suffed eggs because if features eggs stuffed with tuna.

Boil a dozen eggs. Slice in half and mix yolks with:

    1 drained can tuna
    2 T. sherry
    1/2 cup mayonnaise
    1/8 tea. thyme
    1/4 tea. salt
    1/3 cup chopped pecans
    1/8 tea. white pepper
    1 T. chopped parsley

Stuff the eggs with the mixture and put a strip of pimento across the top of each one, if you are traveling first cabin.

Oh, yeah, the recipe for:

Pike Place Spoon Cheese

Go to the Pike Place Market in Seattle and buy some spoon cheese.
And pick up a six-pack of Gusto Beer, while you're there. You only pass this way once.

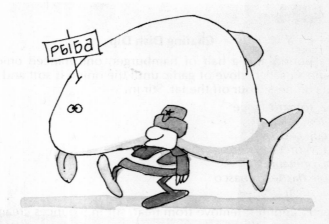

It was at a post-game reception in Seattle for the touring Russian National hockey team. The Soviet skaters hadn't yet arrived but the Totems were there, with their wives, and they walked around the buffet, sniffing it and inspecting it as though it were a whale, beached in the middle of the Hilton Banquet Room.

With a bow toward U.S.-Soviet relations, the kitchen staff had gone heavy on the cold fish and caviar in the impressive display of hors d'oeuvres.

"Wow, this looks great," one of the Totem wives enthused, advancing toward the spread.

"Yeah," admitted another pert young thing, who already had inspected the layout. "But there's nothing to eat!"

Clearly, she was a neophyte, as free-loaders go. The unwritten code of the corps specifies that you consume anything that looks expensive, whether you like it or not.

Never mind that an open-faced caviar sandwich is really a nest of unhatched fish eggs. You eat them anyway, because they cost eleventeen dollars an ounce or something. And make your move toward the little black ones first, because they cost more.

You can then proceed on down the price scale through the crab legs (eat a lot of crab legs), the tiny poached oysters, meanwhile advancing obliquely toward the marinated jumbo prawns.

And then if it is ever your turn to kick through with a spread, emphasize something like gingered meatballs, sherried mushrooms and $2.57 worth of assorted Danish cheeses.

Damn the expense, because they taste good enough to eat.

Gingered Meatballs

3 lbs. ground beef
2 chopped onions
1/2 cup flour
2 cups bread crumbs
2 eggs
2 minced cloves garlic

Dump the above into a large mixing bowl, and form a million or so walnut-sized meatballs.

In a large skillet or electric frying pan heat to boiling three cups water mixed with three beef bouillon cubes, four tablespoons brown sugar, two tablespoons lemon juice and two teaspoons powdered ginger.

Simmer as many meatballs as the skillet will hold for 15 minutes, turning occasionally. If you have more meatballs waiting to jump in, remove the first batch to a warm place while you cook the rest in the broth.

When the balls have all been simmered 15 minutes, mix some flour with some of the ginger sauce in a cup, then stir back into the pan and simmer to thicken sauce slightly.

Dump all the meatballs into a chafing or warming dish, pour the sauce over the top and run it out to the table before one of the guests gets the idea he needs a second drink. If you still can't attract his attention away from the booze, try some:

Sherried Mushrooms

You can use the whole, canned mushrooms. Drain each big, eight-ounce can and dump the mushrooms into a skillet with 1/2 cup butter and 2/3 cup golden sherry. Let this burble around at medium low heat for about 20 minutes, stirring frequently, until the mushrooms are coated and the sauce reduced.

Sprinkle with chopped chives and serve hot with toothpicks.

Oh yeah, the Danish cheese goes on the crackers and if you cover them all up, it will be obvious to your guests that there simply wasn't room for caviar, crab legs and prawns.

I've gotta admit I had a few false starts, before discovering this foolproof recipe for baked bread.

My first few encounters with dough, in virtually any form, did not prove eminently successful. After about the third flogging the dough turned an unhealthy shade of gray, emitted a little sigh, and just seemed to give up.

Actually, one batch turned out all right, when fully baked, although I had not originally intended to manufacture a five-pound door stop.

Then I discovered this foolproof recipe. Two recipes, actually. And you may be surprised to learn they work equally well for fried doughnuts.

First take one (1) Ford Galaxy, point it toward Renton, continue on the Maple Valley road to Black Diamond, turn right down the hill, and purchase two loaves of fresh bread and a dozen doughnuts from the nice lady at the bakery.

The alternate recipe entails driving to Issaquah, taking a hard right, continuing on to Black Diamond, etc. etc.

If it's a nice day, I suggest you drive over to the Green River Gorge to eat your doughnuts, but save some of the bread for supper.

However if you don't live in the Seattle area, or have a hankering for a pizza, you're in trouble. You don't want my recipe for pizza dough, which has been unanimously condemned by the American Dental Society.

I suggest you sneak down to the store and purchase (A) a loaf of frozen bread dough or (B) a box of Pillsbury hot roll mix.

If you've got all day to let the frozen dough thaw and rise, according to the instructions on the wrapper, you'll have ample dough for one large pizza. The hot roll mix, prepared according to the packaged instructions, will give you enough dough for a pizza and a half, so figure that one out. (If you like a thin crust, omit the yeast, which comes in a separate envelope.

Pizza Topping

1 large onion
1 large green pepper
1 can tomato sauce
1 can tomato paste
5 cloves garlic
¾ teaspoon oregano
¼ teaspoon paprika
  dash of cayenne
¼ teaspoon Tabasco
½ teaspoon lemon juice
2 tablespoons parmesan cheese
1 tomato
½ lb. hot Italian sausage
12 ounces mozzarella cheese

Saute the chopped onion in some oil. Add the diced green pepper and when these vegetables are soft dump in the tomato sauce and tomato paste (small can of each). Add the garlic, finely minced, the oregano, paprika, cayenne salt, tabasco, lemon juice and parmesan cheese. Plop the tomato into some boiling water, remove, peel, chop and add to the pot.

Throw the Italian sausage into boiling water, turn heat off and let 'em sit there about 10 or 15 minutes, while the sauce simmers.

Grate the mozzarella cheese. Remove the casings from the sausage and slice.

Then what you do is to spread a thin layer of the sauce over the pizza crust, top with the shredded mozzarella, then with the Italian sausage slices, and pour any leftover sauce over the top.

Toss it into a 350 oven for about 30 minutes.

Goes good with cold beer or hot saki.

"grow" right in your kitchen for less than 20 cents a pound. That food is yogurt . . . and every real devotee of the tasty treat sooner or later develops his or her own special "formula" for brewing up regular batches at home.

Sue Friend—of Cleveland Heights, Ohio —starts by heating a quart of regular or skim milk to a simmer (about 170°F.). Next she pours two or three inches of 130° water into an old portable soft drink cooler. Then she quickly cools the heated milk—also to 130°— by setting the pan in a bigger pot of cold water and stirring it with a thermometer (which she says is easier than using a spoon).

As soon as the milk is down to 130°, Sue

"When the last jar is in place, the hot water should be level with the top of the milk-yogurt mixture in each container. Then it's just a matter of closing the cooler, lid tight and leaving its contents alone for five to seven hours. Once the culture has 'set,' refrigerate the jars until the yogurt is eaten."

Sue claims that her method works every time for her . . . but, as I mentioned above, there's as many schools of thought on yogurt incubation as there are people making the healthful treat. I, for instance, always like to stir three or four drops of pure vanilla flavoring into my batches at the time I add the starter culture to the milk. It gives the finished yogurt a brighter, more "American" taste.

For a 4-page leaflet that contains several other basic yogurt recipes, send 10 cents and a stamped, self-addressed long envelope in care of this newspaper to the Mother Earth News, Dept. SPI, Box 957, Des Moines, Iowa 50304. Ask for Reprint No. 117, "Yogurt."

Tuna Pizza

1 onion
1/4 cup catsup
1/2 tea. salt
1 tea. oregano
1 can drained tuna
1 can tomato sauce
1/2 tea. pepper
1/3 tea. garlic powder
1/4 lb. fresh mushrooms
3/4 pound mozzarella or jack cheese

Saute the chopped onion in oil in a saucepan until golden. Add the tomato sauce, the catsup and seasonings. Let it simmer for about 10 minutes.

Slice the mushrooms and saute briefly in another pan. Grate the cheese and drain the tuna.

Spread the dough thinly over one large, two small or four bitty pans, which have been lightly greased, pinching a small rim around the edge.

Add half the cheese, pour on the sauce, add the remainder of the cheese and top with chunks of tuna and the sauteed mushrooms.

Fling it into a 450 oven and cook for about 20 minutes.

Italian Sausage Pizza

Prepare dough as before and spread out over greased pan, or pans.

Open a small can of tomato sauce and spread evenly over the dough. Remove the sausage from the casings of two hot Italian sausage links and divide the meat in pinches, to cover the top of the pizza. Sprinkle with one teaspoon of mixed Italian seasonings.

Grate some mozzarella cheese (or any leftover cheese in the refrigerator, for that matter) and sprinkle evenly over the top. At this point feel free to clean out the frig completely, adding a few anchovies here, a couple of chopped olives there, etc.

Cook for 15 minutes in a 500 oven, remove, cut into wedges, return to oven for three minutes to reheat and firm it up, then serve.

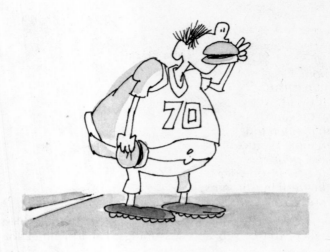

We are raising a generation of giants . . . on 26-cent hamburgers. Dr. Frankenstein messed around with electricity and battery acid. Hitler tried to build a super race on sauerkraut and bockwurst. And all the time the formula was right there before them . . . two buns; a slab of meat, and a pickle.

Our basketball players are seven feet tall, the football stars weigh 300 pounds, and the box boy at the supermarket gets A's in calculus.

Sure, pediatricians push vitamins and food supplements. Parents promote broccoli and are big on granola. But once the teenager of today escapes from this stifling influence, he or she puts away two burgers, a side of fries and grows three more inches.

When you think about it, the diet is perfectly sound. The pickle and the catsup provide all the vegetables a guy should need and the milk shake coats the stomach so that the french fries can't do too much damage.

There's only one thing wrong. Your average 26-cent hamburger has all the flavor of a plastic sponge in a car wash. Unless educated differently, this generation will grow up thinking a chateaubriand is Chevrolet's answer to the Torino, and believing that a sauteed fowl is the equivalent of the slowroller down the third base line.

The solution: Hit 'em where they live. Let them eat hamburgers, but put a little pizazz in their lives.

Double-Headers

2 lbs. ground beef
2 tea. salt
freshly ground pepper
1/2 cup chili sauce
2 T. Worcestershire
1/2 tea. garlic powder
1/2 cups shredded cheddar
1/2 tea. chili powder

Mix the meat, Worcestershire, salt, garlic powder and pepper, form into twice as many balls as you intend to have hamburgers and then flatten them between sheets of waxed paper. Patties should be thin, but even.

In another bowl mix the cheddar, chili sauce and chili powder and use all of this mixture to top half the patties. Use the unadorned patties as lids and press to seal the fillings.

Grill and serve on warm, buttered buns.

Chili Burgers

2 lbs. ground beef
1/4 tea. pepper
2 tea. minced onion
4 T. chopped stuffed green olives
1-1/2 tea. salt
1 cup chili sauce
2 tea. chili powder

Mix beef with the salt and pepper, then add chili sauce, minced onion, chili powder and olives. Form into eight patties and grill.

If you use an electric frying pan, cook about five minutes on each side. If you're barbecuing over a hot fire, about four minutes on a side should be sufficient, because you want the burgers to be moist and flavorful inside . . . so that they'll taste like the 59-cent hefty burgers.

What's that? We need a vegetable to balance the meal?

OK; serve a slice of onion on the side, if you're really a nutrition freak.

Winter days, in Seattle, come in two shades, gray or blue. And the grays far outnumber the blues. In fact, Mother Nature will some weeks pitch seven straight grays at you, along with a faceful of rain. Your sinuses come under attack from little beasties, there is one teaspoonful of sand under each eyelid and trenchfoot is a real possibility. At that point you need a blue real bad, but had better be willing to settle for a white, by spending the day on the ski slopes, working up an appetite for:

White Sunday Sandwiches

4-5 lbs. lean pork
3/4 tea. liquid smoke
1 sliced onion
2 tea. salt, pepper

The night before you head for the slopes prepare the meat, which will probably be in the form of a pork butt roast. Cut away as much fat as possible and carve pork into small cubes.

Dump one-third of the pork into the bottom of a loaf pan, season with salt, pepper and 1/4 tea. liquid smoke and top with a couple of slices of onion. Add more meat, more seasoning, more onion until you have used everything in three layers. Completely seal the entire pan with a couple of layers of heavy duty aluminum foil and refrigerate.

The next morning, between the moment when you can't find one ski pole and have jammed the zipper on your stretch pants, put the wrapped loaf into a 250 oven.

About 10 hours later, when you're down out of the hills, warm up some hamburger buns and maybe some baked beans, get out the potato chips, and mix together in a saucepan:

1 cup catsup
10 shakes salt
10 grindings pepper
juice of one lemon
10 shakes dried mustard
1/3 cup Worcestershire

Let this simmer for five or 10 minutes while you remove loaf pan from oven, unwrap, and moosh all the pork and juices together with a couple of forks.

Serve the barbecued pork between the heated hamburger buns with a gravy boat of the warm sauce on the side and check the paper to see if there's a special on stretch pants maybe a size or two larger.

As long as you persist in spending a third of your time in bed, it wouldn't hurt to have some interesting dreams.

Obviously, determination isn't enough. You might put in a reservation for Senta Berger and instead find yourself swimming the English Channel with a duck on your head. But a little informed preparation can't hurt.

For instance, you're going to get nowhere if you insist upon belting yourself with graham crackers and milk before you turn in. What kind of excitement are you going to generate with graham crackers and milk? If you're lucky, you'll get stuck in an elevator for six hours with a lifesize plastic Popeye.

In fact it might be wise to give milk a wide berth altogether, especially if it's warm. It often induces a deep coma, and discourages dreaming.

What you have to do is light a little fire in the boiler, maybe with a cold baked bean sandwich on pumpernickle, or possibly a leftover anchovy pizza.

Listed on the following page are a couple of added suggestions which also happen to taste good, a definite plus for midnight snackers.

There is one thing you should know about these sandwich recipes in advance. They contain onions.

Onion is excellent dream material. Unfortunately, if you share your bed with a friend you are going to blow him (or her) clear off the Beautyrest with your first contented sigh. If you snore a lot, your roommate is going to suspect that a crop-duster is spraying mace during low runs across the bedroom ceiling.

But, of course, if your marriage is built upon soggy graham crackers, it won't last long, anyway. Go ahead and grind up the midnight material for what you could call a Senta-Cheese-Berger.

Senta-Cheese-Berger

Peel and quarter a large Bermuda onion. Toss it into a food chopper (or blender) with one pound of sharp cheddar cheese and enough mayonnaise (quite a lot of mayonnaise, in fact) to make a spread.

Taste the mixture and if it doesn't lift the lid of your skull, you might add some salt and pepper to taste.

What you do next is make some toast. When browned lightly on both sides, spread the cheese-onion mixture on one side, slide the toast under the broiler briefly, remove when bubbly, sprinkle with paprika, and eat.

The leftover spread can be saved in a refrigerator crock for future nightmares.

Another Nocturnal Adventure

For each sandwich, cut one slice of bacon in small pieces and fry until crisp. Remove from pan and toss a generous slice of Bermuda onion, separated into rings, into the bacon fat. When the onion is soft and translucent, gather it into a little nest in the frying pan, add the crisp bacon and break an egg over the top.

Deftly pluck the yolk with a fork, top with a slice of cheese, and sprinkle with salt and pepper. Cook, covered, over low heat until egg is done, the cheese is melted, and the covers have been turned down in the bedroom.

Obviously, if you are a two-sandwich man, you'll begin with two pieces of bacon, two slices of onion, two eggs, and etc., etc.

If you are a three or four-sandwich man, you will also soon be a hermit.

But, wow, what crazy dreams!

Soup and Chili

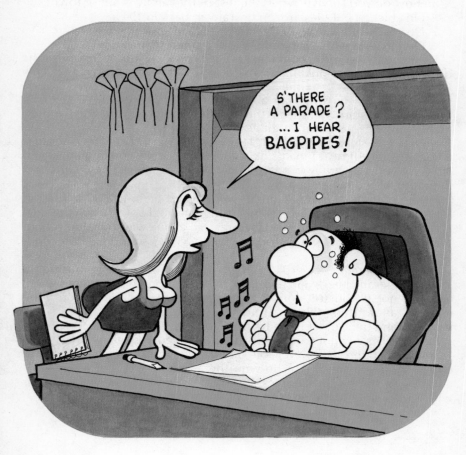

So how do you survive, when the rest of the family is out of town?

— On chicken pot pies, frozen on Taiwan back in 1949?

— Do you heat up a can of beenie-weenie in your shaving water?

— Or make-do with a can of beer and a gingersnap?

It's not necessary. You could just as easily pick up your secretary, or the divorcee down the block, and invest in a saddle of lamb at that new French restaurant.

Of course, if your wife hears about your fun night out, the chances are excellent that you will spend the remainder of your life surviving on frozen pies, beenie-weenies, gingersnaps and beer.

Myself, I like to whip up about 11 pounds of Son O'Gun Stew, because it contains lots of neat innards like lamb kidneys. Try cooking up a lamb kidney when the family is around, and minor relatives begin clutching their throats and falling heavily to the floor.

Eleven pounds of Son O'Gun Stew, reheated periodically, will last at least until Friday, with maybe some instant mashed potatoes on the side.

A cast-iron pot of baked beans will also go a long way, but along about Wednesday afternoon your stomach will begin to sound like a second-hand bagpipe.

And then there is a casserole built around hard-boiled eggs, mushroom soup; parmesan cheese and about six pounds of onions. That goes good, too, but not if you still consider your secretary a viable option. (The reason I can say things like that and get away with it is that I don't have a secretary and the closest thing to it is a copyboy with a mustache.)

Bean soup is a winner, but there are those bagpipes again.

Split pea soup is thus a reliable alternative, with fewer harmful side-effects. And you can jazz it up with the addition of 3/4 of a pound of chorizos, or hot Italian sausages. It should last most of the week. If your wife is suspicious and won't leave, it'll serve six at one meal, generously.

So Long Soup

Buy a pound bag of split peas, wash them two or three times, drain and toss into a large soup kettle. Cut 3/4 lb. sausage links in half and toss into the pot, along with a sliced stalk of celery, a chopped onion, a mashed clove of garlic, one teaspoon of basil and some chopped up parsley.

Add nine cups of hot water, bring to a boil, then reduce heat and cook covered for two hours at a low simmer. Remove sausages, cut in half-inch slices and return to the pot.

Fling in four sliced carrots, two cubed potatoes, a few grindings of pepper and about two teaspoons of salt, or whatever tastes fair.

Cook over medium heat another 30 minutes, and you are set for the week, although you may have to thin it out periodically with a cup of hot water, maybe with a chicken bouillon cube tossed in for good measure.

Of course, if you are partial to bagpipes:

Beanareeno Zoop

1-1/2 lbs. assorted dried beans
2 chopped onions
1 T. salt
ham bone, or hocks
2 chicken bouillon cubes
generous pinches sage and thyme
1 diced carrot
3 cloves garlic
3-1/2 quarts water
1/2 cup catsup
1 cup potato buds

Soak the beans overnight, drain and wash. Put some cooking oil in a pot and saute the chopped onions until golden. Meanwhile dice the carrot. Peel the garlic cloves and mash them up in the same dish with the salt.

Dump everything into the pot . . . the hot water, beans, garlic, the ham bone, bouillon cubes, instant potatoes, the catsup, carrot and spices.

Simmer, slowly, for four hours. Let the soup cool overnight, remove the ham from the bone and discard the latter. Skim the fat off the top, reheat, taste to see if it needs more salt (I think it does) and serve with lots of crusty French bread.

If you eat it all up you can have a gingersnap for dessert.

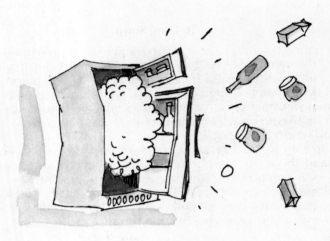

Chances are that you've never had a fire deputy rummage through your refrigerator for evidence. But I suspect the Fire Department frowns upon partially-filled bottles of wine.

Left unattended in the refrigerator, a half-filled bottle of Chianti is a smoldering time bomb. I think it's like gasoline fumes in the bilge of a boat. The little light goes on in your refrigerator. And Powie!

Well, no, I haven't actually seen a refrigerator blow up, and lack any first-person testimony. But I did hear a muffled explosion a few weeks ago. Sounded like Beaujolais in a Kelvinator, to me.

The reason one of my refrigerators has never blown up is that we run a taut kitchen. You won't find any oily rags in the cellar or half-filled bottles of wine in the kitchen. If, by necessity, a jug must be uncorked and three tablespoons removed for sauteed chicken livers, the rest of the wine is disposed of as quickly as possible, and certainly in the same day.

The trick, then, is to assemble a file of recipes calling for miniscule amounts of wine. A burgandy beef stew requiring a full fifth of vino should be quickly destroyed, because it offers the cook no reward.

The recipe on the next page is a distinct improvement, since it calls for less than half a bottle. The remainder may be chilled for an apertif, but don't let it sit in the refrigerator too long, or you'll be picking pieces of your Frost King out of the ceiling.

Gruyere Onion Soup

Recipes for onion soup can be prepared in 15 minutes or 15 hours, depending upon whether you begin with an envelope, or with three pounds of beef brisket and cracked goat shins. This one falls somewhere between the two extremes.

To serve four, begin with two cans of beef stock, which will shortly be made palatable.

First, lightly brown two quartered onions and one quartered carrot in two tablespoons butter, which have been melted in a saucepan. Add 3/4 cup white wine and boil until it is reduced. Stir in the two cans of stock, two peeled garlic cloves, a handful of parsley, two celery tops and 1/2 teaspoon of thyme. Bring to a boil, reduce heat and simmer 30 minutes. Once you have strained the stock, you are ready for an assault on the onions.

Saute two thinly sliced onions until golden, in three tablespoons of butter. Stir in a tablespoon of flour, add a cup of the white wine and the beef stock. Toss in a pinch of nutmeg and salt and pepper to taste.

Cover and simmer over very low heat for an hour. Near the end of the hour trim the crust from four slices of bread. Fry these bread squares in a buttered frying pan until brown and crisp. Set aside. Grate a quarter pound of Gruyere cheese, and set aside.

When soup is ready, add two tablespoons of grated Gruyere cheese and stir in.

Ladle soup into four generous ovenproof bowls. Place one square fried bread in each. Top the bread with the remaining cheese. Place the bowls in the oven, under broiler, until cheese melts (just a couple of minutes) and serve steaming hot.

Gadzooks, I detect a rumbling in the Cold Spot. You didn't forget the leftover wine!!!

For quite awhile, they had me confused, but I am beginning to detect a pattern behind the rating system for contemporary movies. G means the featured actor is a bear cub. And X means my wife doesn't want to see it. I'm still working on GP and R.

Obviously, some sort of rating system should guide our culinary adventures, particularly in the area of food described as piquant.

One recent summer I encountered a restaurant that rated its Indian curries from one to five stars. However, the difference proved to be that of biting down on a cherry bomb (one star) or a stick of dynamite (the beef vindaloo). And that's really not any choice at all.

A lot of Spanish and Mexican food is also piquant, but I have fortunately evolved a five-star rating system which is semi-foolproof. Say you're eating a bowl of soup, containing a questionable measure of cayenne.

If you can finish the bowl of soup before you have to blow your nose, it rates one star. Two honks, two stars. See, how easy? A four means you have to reach for the handkerchief four or more times. A "five" means you developed a bad case of hiccups with the first spoonful.

The shrimp soup which follows rates one star, which means that even minor relatives can consume it without breaking into uncontrollable sobs.

The research into this dish began in an attempt to duplicate the shrimp soup served by the late Ramon Palaez at the Copacabana Cafe, in Seattle's Pike Place Market.

This is an excellent substitute, although it isn't the same as the Copacabana version. Repeated trips confirmed without a doubt that Ramon served a genuine "four."

One Star Shrimp Soup

2 T. olive oil
2 cloves garlic
3 T. tomato sauce
1/2 cup chopped carrots
1/2 tea. marjoram
2 dried chili peppers
2 eggs
2 chopped onions
6 cups boiling water
1/2 cup frozen green peas
2 tea. salt
4 small potatoes
4 oz. cream cheese
1 cup milk

And, ohhh, about $1.50 worth of those little shrimp looking up at you there from the supermarket tray.

Heat the oil in your soup kettle and add the onions, chopped, and the two peeled cloves of garlic. Saute them over low heat for 10 minutes, stirring, then remove and discard the garlic buds.

Dump in the water, tomato sauce, peas, carrots, marjoram and the potatoes, peeled and diced. Put the salt and the two dried chili peppers in a mortar and grind them thoroughly with a pestle, then dump the mixture into the pot and cook briskly for 20 minutes.

Mash the cream cheese and add to the soup. Toss in the shrimp and cook, stirring occasionally, for another 10 minutes. Beat the eggs to a froth, add at least a cup of the hot soup, stirring. Then pour this egg-soup mixture back into the pot, still stirring. Add the cup of milk and reheat, but don't boil.

If you are interested in something more like a three or a four-star soup, just double the number of chili peppers, but don't feed more than a bowlful to nursing infants.

If you're too lazy to cook your own shrimp soup, Ramon Palaez' son and daughters have reopened the Copacabana and have managed to duplicate most of his unwritten recipes.

I checked out their shrimp soup not long ago, consumed a bowl with gusto and rated it a "one" on the handkersniff chart. However, a couple of dollops of the chili sauce they serve on the side converted it to a "four" real quick.

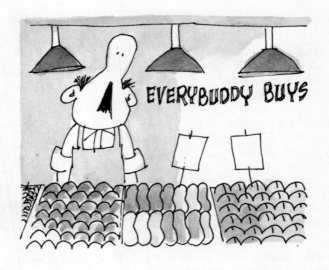

In the world of commerce, the Pike Place Market occupies a position as a mixed bag.

You can buy chicken livers and pig tails, leather belts and second-hand shoes, Wilkie buttons and hippie beads, incense and radishes, turnip greens and peace posters, cotton candy and cracked crab, a plate of fried oysters or a sack of deep fried chicken wings.

Don't mention it. I get hungry just thinking about a sack of deep fried chicken wings. "You want some salt and a paper napkin?" she asks. (Do I want them salted, with a paper napkin!)

Don't mention spoon cheese, either. If you mention spoon cheese, I'll buy a half-pound and then I might not have enough change left for the chicken wings.

That's the trouble with the Pike Place Market. The place is long on nummies. For example, you should never visit the Pike Place Market without buying some deep fried chicken wings at the corner stand, a half-pound of spoon cheese at Brehm's Delicatessen, a bowl of shrimp soup at the Copacabana Cafe, some hot dogs and cold cuts from the Bavarian Meat Market, a sack of orange-spiced tea from the Specialty Spice Shop, a mug of Danish beer from the Athenian Cafe and a pound of freshly grated Parmesan cheese from DeLaurenti's Italian Grocery.

What do you do with a pound of freshly grated Parmesan cheese from De Laurenti's Italian Grocery? Well, you could whip up a kettle of:

Pike Place Soup

On a leisurely stroll of the street-level stalls, select:

1 onion
1 small zucchini
2 stalks celery
1 tomato
2 carrots
2 T. parsley

Peel; chop and then cook vegetables slowly until softened in two tablespoons of olive oil. (Of course, you put the olive oil in the soup kettle first. Scheeeez!)

Add to the kettle 1-1/2 or 2 quarts of water and five beef bouillon cubes. (You can use beef stock instead, if you happen to have some stored away in your freezer. But you don't. I looked. Your freezer is filled with popsicles and Mexican TV dinners.) For seasoning, toss in one teaspoon of salt, a few grindings of fresh pepper and 1/2 tea. thyme.

Simmer for 30 minutes, ladle into bowls, serve, and pass around a generous bowl of the freshly grated Parmesan. (If it isn't freshly grated, you're on your own, Leonard.)

Orrrr, for a simpler luncheon soup you might consider:

Chicken and Egg Soup

To four cups of hot bouillon, add two tablespoons of minced parsley and two tablespoons of freshly grated Parmesan. Taste, and add salt and pepper as needed.

While the bouillon is heating to a boil, whip two eggs until frothy. While the soup comes to a slow boil, pour the egg into the pan in a slow dribble, stirring constantly.

Lower heat, continue stirring for another five minutes, and serve, maybe with some crackers, a half pound of spoon cheese, a few deep fried chicken wings . . .

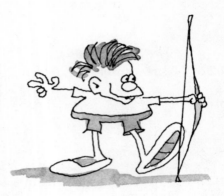

As a traditional Day-After-Christmas dish, you might give some consideration to a recipe the children will probably detest. I mean, you've been pampering the little beggars for about two weeks, stuffing them with candy canes, cracked nuts, fruit cake, marshmallow reindeer and some of that weird dried fruit which Uncle Elmo persists in mailing up from Palm Desert.

You've been fretting over whether Little Gloria would rather have a doll that burps or one that wets. You've equipped Junior with a bow and arrow that is going to shorten the life expectancy of the neighbor's cat by three and one-half years. You've filled the stocking with 492 objects that a baby can swallow at its peril.

And then you asked, "Did you have a good Christmas?" suggesting that the dwarfs in your house grade your largesse on a scale of one to ten.

Just to put things back in proportion, one day after Christmas when they sit down to lunch or dinner, you might snarl:

"Here's a bowl of curried turkey soup. Eat it or I'll belt you on the ear."

Some of the children will claim that their skulls are on fire, but anyone past puberty should benefit from a steaming bowl of the soup. For one thing, it clears your sinuses in a jiffy. For another thing, it provides an excuse for disposing of that skeleton, after it has been staring out of the refrigerator at you for a week or so. And it is certainly superior to your average bowl of turkey soup, which just lies there looking up at you.

32

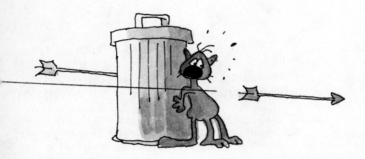

Curried Turkey Soup

The day before you plan to alienate your offspring, cover the earthly remains of the bird with two inches of water in a large pot. Toss in two tablespoons of salt and simmer for five or 10 minutes, skimming the scum as it rises. (If you didn't get an electric scum skimmer for Christmas you can use a spoon.) Toss in two peeled onions stuck with two cloves, two chopped carrots, two chopped stalks of celery, some chopped-up parsley and one-quarter teaspoon of sage.

Simmer slowly, uncovered, for three hours, adding water as needed. Strain the liquid into a bowl or pitcher and refrigerate. Remove the turkey from the bones and set aside.

Next day, skim the fat off the chilled stock and reheat.

Melt four tablespoons butter in another large saucepan. Stir in two or three teaspoons of curry powder and cook slowly for a minute. Add one chopped onion and cook, occasionally stirring, until limp and golden. Stir in six tablespoons flour and cook another couple of minutes.

Remove this pan from the heat and slowly pour the heated stock atop the curried onions, beating as you pour with a wire whip. Return to heat, continue stirring, then add instant mashed potato buds to the soup, a spoonful at a time, until it is as thick as you prefer. Taste and see if it needs a teaspoon of salt. Toss in the turkey meat, maybe some chopped chives, heat, serve, and stare sternly at the first kid that complains.

As you probably recall, meatball soup evolved as the commemorative dish to mark the lifting of The Great Beef Price Freeze in 1973.

You bake a turkey at Thanksgiving, braise a ham for Easter, and eat meatball soup to celebrate the week of the big beef thaw. It has been ever so.

Maybe it is considered the traditional feast because the hot soup speeds the thawing process. Or maybe it was the favorite dish of Vilhjalmur Stefansson, the man who ended the first national beef freeze. Appropriately enough, Vilhjalmur Stefansson was an Arctic explorer.

You may not know that in the early 1900s, beef was suspect as an article of diet. That's what my encyclopedia says. Eating meat more than twice a week was supposed to promote rheumatism, harden the old arteries and weaken the kidneys.

Actually, it doesn't do any of these things. Eating beef merely puts a fast leak in your wallet.

Vilhjalmur Stefansson was the guy responsible for the education of a nation. He had wandered all over the Arctic Circle, swallowing seal eyes, munching blubber, carving up caribou steaks and avoiding peas and carrots like a plague. And he challenged medical science to find something wrong with his kidneys.

In 1928 he was examined and re-examined at Bellevue Hospital in New York. At the conclusion of the tests, all the doctors ran home and thawed out some ground round for meatball soup. They should have suspected the truth before, being scientific men. After all, their laboratory rats ate lettuce three times a day, but didn't have what you would really call colossal prospects for the future.

Undoubtedly you have your own traditional family recipe for meatball soup, handed down generation by generation. This one uses two cans of potato soup, some carrots and onions but leaves out the seal eyes.

Traditional Meatball Soup

Mix one pound of ground beef in a big bowl with a cup of soft bread crumbs, 1/4 cup of minced onion, 1 tea. salt, 1/4 cup of milk, a tea. Worcestershire sauce and one beaten egg. Form into walnut-sized meatballs and place on a large flat pan, which has been covered with waxed paper. Refrigerate.

In a large pot combine:

2 cups water
4 sliced carrots
1 onion peeled and coarsely chopped
2 T. margarine
1-1/2 tea. salt

Bring to a slow simmer, cover and cook 15 minutes. Add two cans of undiluted cream of potato soup and one teaspoon of dill weed. Reheat, but do not boil.

Add the meatballs, one at a time, cover and simmer slowly for 20 minutes. Generously serves four adults — or 12 laboratory animals.

Steak Soup

Don't get scared off. All we're talking about is about four of those skinny little breakfast steaks, which I think maybe the butcher cuts off an eye of round.

Cut the meat into thin strips. Then chop up four green onions, mince a clove of garlic and toss everything into a pot along with 1-1/2 pints of chicken stock, two tablespoons soy sauce, and maybe a smidgen of salt and pepper, to taste.

Toss into the pot 12 ounces fresh bean sprouts, let simmer 15 minutes, and serve.

Scipio's Soup

2 T. cooking oil
2 lbs. stew meat
mashed clove garlic
1 green pepper
5 cups water
1/8 tea. pepper
1/8 tea. Tabasco
2 T. margarine
2 chopped onions
1 T. paprika
2 tomatoes
2 tea. salt
1 tea. caraway seed
2 potatoes

Heat two tablespoons of oil in large stew pot. Cut meat into bite-sized hunks and brown, a handful at a time, then set aside in a warm place.

Pour off the oil and toss the two tablespoons of margarine into the same pot. Add two chopped onions and the garlic and saute over low heat until soft. Stir in the paprika, return the meat to the pot along with the green pepper (seeded and cut into strips), the tomatoes (peeled, seeded and chopped), the water, salt, pepper, caraway seeds and Tabasco.

Bring everything to a boil, lower heat and simmer, covered, for two hours. Add the potatoes, peeled and cut into large hunks, cook for another 30 minutes, and serve.

Canal Chowder

1 large onion
2 cloves garlic
1 cup water
1 tea. paprika
salt
1 lb. shrimp, or less

1 cup margarine
2 large potatoes
1 chicken bouillon cube
1 quart milk
pepper

Thinly slice onion, mince the garlic and saute in the melted margarine. Cook gently in a large sauce pan until the onion is translucent, but not brown.

Add the potatoes, thinly sliced, water, bouillon, paprika, salt and pepper, to taste. Cook slowly until the potatoes are quite tender, then add milk and reheat (but don't boil).

Add cooked, cleaned shrimp, let them swim around in the chowder for about five minutes, then serve, maybe with some cheddar cheese biscuits.

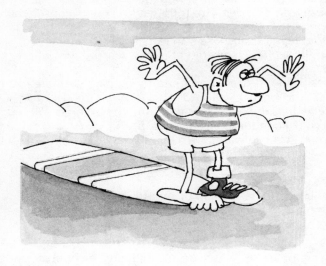

Whatdaya mean, you've never heard of the World's Chili Championship at Terlingua, Texas? Well, certainly you're familiar with J. J. Moon, the world's greatest surfer. Like the World's Chili Championship, he was the promotional creation of a guy named Bill Doner.

"We had bumper stickers, sweatshirts, and a 1,000-member J. J. Moon Fan Club," Doner remembers fondly. "We got a two-page spread in Life (and may have killed that publication). We said he was the world's greatest surfer because he had 11 toes. See, the only surfer in the world who could Hang 11. When he went to the beach he wore a tennis shoe on one foot, so nobody knew for sure . ."

Doner brought Texas chili to the Northwest, where he now promotes motor racing. Fortunately, he left J. J. Moon down south, where his single tennis shoe is now probably leaving forlorn tracks on some remote beach.

Personally, I like his recipe for Texas chili, although I admit that it makes my ear lobes ache. It is powerful. If the Ski Patrol carried it in steaming jugs, they would never have to pack anybody down the hill on a stretcher. One bite will clear a severe head cold. A bowlful, formed into a poultice, will likely cure pneumonia.

Unfortunately, Texas chili also makes children scream and weak women sob uncontrollably. So I hereby offer a satisfactory substitute. Texas chili is hotter, but this just may be gooder.

Cascade Crest Chili

Texas chili is cooked for something like six days and served up with a sprinkling of gun powder. The following recipe is considerably quicker and will provide three giant servings or four average bowls. You might want to double it, because it's also excellent when reheated.

Mash three peeled cloves of garlic in a teaspoon of salt. Hey, that's a heckuva start!

Heat a tablespoon of salad oil in a frying pan, crumble in a pound of beef chuck and brown well. Add 1/2 cup chopped celery, a chopped onion, the garlic-salt paste and saute until the onion is soft.

Stir in a can of condensed tomato soup, a 15-ounce can of kidney beans in their liquid, 3/4 cup water, 1 tea. paprika, 3 or 4 teaspoons chili powder and 1 teaspoon allspice.

Pour everything into a casserole, cover and bake 30 to 45 minutes in a 350-degree oven.

Remove lid, sprinkle 1/2 cup of shredded cheddar cheese over the top and return to oven until cheese melts.

Chili-con-Golli

This is a recipe for those who think chili must be built around dried hot chili peppers. Use two of the peppers if you have a low boiling point, or six peppers if you like to weep and blow your nose a lot.

> 1 to 1-1/2 lbs. ground meat
> 6 cloves garlic
> 1 can tomato sauce
> 2 to 6 chili peppers
> 1 tea. ground cumin
> 1 onion
> 28-oz. can tomatoes
> 1-1/2 T. salt
> 1 T. caraway seeds
> medium can kidney beans

Melt two tablespoons of lard in your skillet. Add the ground meat, in bits, the chopped onion and the minced cloves of garlic. Worry everything around in the pan with a wooden spoon until the meat has lost its redness and the onion is soft.

If you have a blender, smash up the canned tomatoes this way and add to the pan, along with the tomato sauce, the caraway, cumin and the chili peppers, which you have previously worked over, with the salt, in a mortar and pestel.

Simmer 3 to 4 hours covered, add the can of kidney beans (a larger can, if you have a larger family) and simmer an hour longer, with the lid off the last 20 minutes, if it's still a little soupy.

Seafood

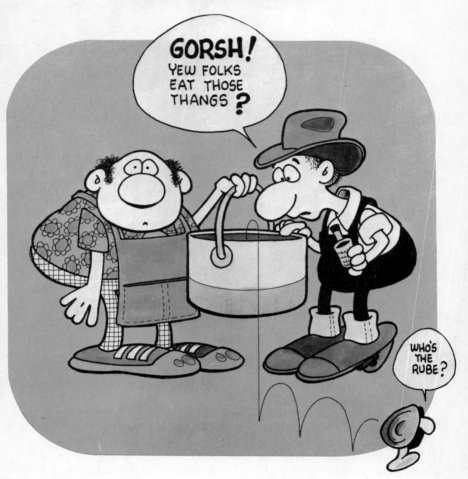

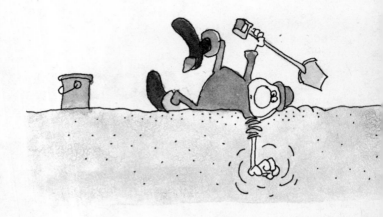

It begins as an act of kindness, an expression of charity for the less fortunate. You're visited by some friends or relatives from the great heartland of America, and you decide to enrich their lives in some small manner.

Clams!

That's it! Serve 'em a pot of steamed clams ... those little blue- and gray-babies from Hood Canal, some melted butter, a cup of clam nectar and a basketful of French bread. A little bit of Puget Sound, in a pot.

And then you place the pot on the table.

"Hoo, boy, whada we got here?" the husband shouts exuberantly, and then begins to swallow nervously. "Are they dead or am I supposed to kill 'em with this cocktail pick?"

His wife just sits there, transfixed. For the same effect you could have served up John the Baptist's tonsils, en brochette.

And they spend the next 33 quiet minutes rearranging clam shells on their plates.

"Hey, this sure is great French bread!" the husband finally booms out, gnawing off another noisy hunk.

"Feel free to dip it in your clam nectar," you suggest, helpfully.

And he drops the French bread heavily to his plate, his mouth ajar just at the thought.

So much for that culinary adventure. Accept it. Some people go through life satisfactorily stuffing themselves with goulash and meat loaf.

Which leaves us with a question of social conscience: Should we let them?

Maybe not. It just might be possible to sneak up on them, with a fantastic dish like:

40

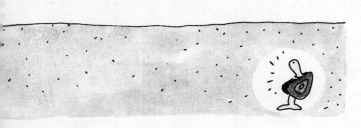

Walla Walla Clams

Actually, the clams aren't from Walla Walla. But the pork can be. You'll need about two pounds of it — lean, boneless pork cut into half-inch cubes.

Marinate the pork cubes for about half a day in a mixture of two cups dry white wine, a tablespoon of paprika, pepper and three garlic cloves which have been mashed with one teaspoon of salt.

You'll need two pounds of clams and if you buy them at your local fish market you need follow only this simple guide: If their tongues are hanging out, let 'em commit suicide in somebody else's pot. If the clams are almost tightly closed, it means that they are in superb condition, or filled with sand.

Drain the pork, pat it lovingly with a paper towel, but save the marinade.

Heat two tablespoons lard in large pan until it begins to smoke. Saute pork cubes over high heat, stirring frequently, until nicely browned all over. Pour in the marinade and boil vigorously for five minutes. Get all the brown nummies off the bottom of the pan with a wooden spoon, while stirring.

Toss in the clams and keep pan over high heat until the clam shells open. Slursh mixture around for a minute with the wooden spoon and serve with seasoned rice and French bread.

Serves about six Puget Sounders or 123 visitors from Muncie, Indiana.

Think about it real hard. What could possibly taste, or smell, better than a mess of sauteed onions?

Give up? A mess of sauteed onions generously flecked with minced garlic.

Okay, next question. What could possibly taste better than sauteed onions and garlic?

Well, how about a spicy chorizo sausage, which contains onions and garlic and about 92 spices. Is it possible anything could taste better than some chorizo sausages sizzling slowly in a skillet?

Yes, as a matter of fact. Steamed clams taste even better. Because steamed Puget Sound clams, performing a lazy backstroke in a warm pond of neclar and white wine, taste better than anything in the civilized world. (That takes care of all clam-haters!) But wait, wait.

What would you think if I told you I know a recipe which contains copious onions and garlic and chorizos and wine and clams? You'd probably think either one of two things:

— The man has discovered the formula for ambrosia!

— Or, that sounds like a real gut-buster.

Actually, both of the above are true.

You would naturally not serve it as a substitute for Gerber's Carrot Puree.

If you are due for open-heart surgery the first thing in the morning, it would probably be unwise to put away two bowls of the spiced clams as a midnight snack.

And a person headed for a final Red Cross examination on mouth-to-mouth resuscitation might hold off on the onion and garlic until the grades are in.

But for those of us with stout hearts, and strong stomachs, there is nothing like an occasional:

Puget Sound Gut-Buster

2 onions
dried red peppers
black pepper
1 tea. paprika
1-1/2 cups tomatoes
2 to 3 lbs. little neck clams (to serve four)
3/4 lb. chorizo or hot Italian sausage
2 cloves garlic
1/2 cup olive oil
1/2 cup parsley
1/2 cup dry white wine

Thinly slice the peeled onions. Peel the garlic cloves. Chop the garlic up fine with from one to four red peppers, depending upon your tolerance to dried fire. Be sure to chop the peppers into tiny bits, otherwise one of the flakes will lodge in your throat and cause you to go "AAAgggghhhhh!"

Remove the sausage from the casings. Crumble half of it into a sieve, immerse in boiling water for a minute, remove and dry, and repeat process with the rest of the sausage meat. Discard the water.

Pour the oil into a large pot over medium heat. Stir-cook the onions until soft. Add the sausage meat and continue stir-cooking for three minutes, or until meat has lost all of its redness.

Add the chopped garlic and red pepper, a few grindings of black pepper, the parsley, paprika, wine and the tomatoes, which you should now chop up with a wooden spoon.

Bring to a boil and cook, stirring occasionally, until the liquid is slightly reduced.

Toss in the washed clams, cover, and steam 5 to 8 minutes, or until all the clams have opened.

Serve in bowls with lots of crusty French bread on the side, maybe with the rest of that white wine, slightly chilled.

I had it for breakfast, once. I think my stomach gave just the slightest growl, as though to say:

"Thanks! I needed that!"

It is a cruel hoax, perpetuated by some Manhattan magazine picture editors, who think the Radio City ice rink is the fringe of the polar cap. They consider sand something invented to time soft boiled eggs. Strewn along the ground, it becomes a magic carpet for the beach picnic.

Fraud! Webster defines sand as "a loose, granular material resulting from the disintegration of rocks that is used in mortar, glass, abrasives and foundry molds."

Nothing at all about picnics. Because beaches and picnics don't mix. Violate this basic law of nature, and you end up with sand in your bicuspid.

Yet the typical magazine layout shows five bronzed gods and goddesses, stretched out like lizards on hot rocks, sipping frozen daquiris while their jovial chef whips up some Caesar Salad, to go with the roasted kid, turning slowly on the spit.

Enchanted readers, attempting to duplicate this scene, invariably wind up with second degree burns on a thumb and third degree burns on a hot dog. A 40-knot wind invariably roars in from the ocean at cocktail time, it requires 30 minutes and 40 matches to light a beachwood fire, which emits a greasy black smoke at alternating angles. The beans are steaming and speckled with ash when served onto the plate, and are instantly transformed into a glob of congealed abrasives by the Pacific gale.

The only completely contented participant is the guy who grabbed a jug and disappeared under the driftwood.

Moral: Never take your picnic to the beach. Bring the beach to your picnic. A good place to start is Hood Canal, which abounds with oysters, clams, shrimp and an amazing assortment of fish. Grab as many goodies as you can, then run like a bandit for your kitchen, patio or backyard barbecue to construct something like this:

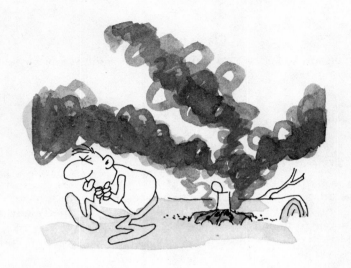

Hood Canal Stew

Into a large kettle deposit a cube of butter, one large chopped onion, two mashed cloves of garlic and some chopped parsley.

Cook until onions are soft, then glunk in a large can of tomatoes, two cups of chicken broth and generous pinches of basil, thyme and oregano. Cover and simmer 30 to 45 minutes.

Pour in a cup and a half of dry white wine and let simmer another 15 minutes. Toss in the fish, cook another 20 minutes and you're in business.

The choice of fish is up to you, your tastes and your good luck, but must include clams and oysters. If it doesn't, I simply won't be responsible.

Try tossing in about three dozen unopened clams, about the same number of oysters which have been unlocked with your oyster knife, and don't forget to include the oyster liquor. Throw in a couple of big handfuls of Hood Canal shrimp if you were able to buy some along the way, or else open a can of inexpensive shrimp pieces. If you caught a fish or two in the canal, cut the meat into big chunks and toss into the pot. A cracked crab wouldn't hurt.

The fish will rub shoulders with the oysters. The clams will open and release their juices with the oyster liquor, the tomatoes, the broth and the wine. Serve with the remaining white wine and French bread.

If you want to consume the feast while seated in junior's sand box, that's your hang-up, not mine.

Clams Camano

To serve four, steam two cups of white rice while you are assembling the following:

4 T. butter
4 lbs. clams
2 cups chicken broth
1 cup white wine
2 cloves garlic
4 T. chopped parsley

Heat the butter in a large, heavy pan. Add the parsley and mashed cloves of garlic and saute one or two minutes. Pour in the chicken broth and wine and bring to a boil. Add the cleaned and brushed clams, cover and steam five to 10 minutes.

Spoon the rice into a soup dish, arrange clams in each bowl and pour the broth over all.

Candlelight Clametti

For a romantic candlelight supper for two, assemble:

2 small cans chopped clams, or equivalent of fresh
1/2 tea. garlic powder
Parmesan cheese
1/2 cup dry white wine
1/2 lb. spaghetti
4 T. butter
1 tea. Italian seasoning
chopped parsley

Melt the butter in a saucepan, add the undrained clams, the wine and the seasonings. Simmer for 20 minutes.

While the clams are absorbing this Italian influence, cook the half-pound of spaghetti in boiling water as directed on the package.

Put a generous portion of cooked spaghetti in each of two deep bowls, top it with a healthy slug (or maybe two or three slugs) of the clam sauce, sprinkle generously with the parsley, and grated Parmesan cheese.

You should have ample spaghetti and sauce for seconds, unless you have something else on your schedule.

Mafia Oysters

Preheat oven to 450 while you are buttering a large ovenproof platter.

Chop two cloves of garlic and cook-stir for a few seconds in four tablespoons of melted butter. Add 1-1/2 cups of fresh bread crumbs and stir-cook until golden. Remove from heat, toss in two tablespoons of chopped parsley.

Spread half of the crumbs over the bottom of the buttered platter. Arrange the oysters on top. (If medium or large oysters are used, chop 'em in half.) Stir three tablespoons of grated Parmesan cheese into remaining crumbs, scatter atop the oysters, dot with butter and cook 10 to 15 minutes until dark golden.

For dessert, you might consider:

Sherried Oysters

Whack up some cornflakes until you are staring at some cornflake crumbs. Spread them out on some waxed paper.

Melt a cube of butter, add one teaspoon of prepared mustard and two tablespoons dry sherry.

Dry oysters, then dunk 'em in the butter mixture, next rolling until covered in the cornflake crumbs.

Place the oysters on the cookie sheet, dribble any remaining butter-sherry mixture over the top and broil in a hot oven about six inches from the flame five to seven minutes total, turning once with a spatula.

Pete Rozelle doesn't know the first thing about sports scheduling.

Neither, for that matter, do the men running the other major league sports.

Because the football teams start messing up the grass during baseball season. The basketball and hockey teams interfere with the football season. And baseball gets in everybody's way.

Those ratty little kids down the block . . . they should be running big league sports. They don't have any problems booking their events into the vacant lot. Oh, there may be some minor scheduling conflicts, but nothing that can't be settled in a fair fight.

Football season starts on the same day the kids are sentenced to school. It continues until the 20 yard line disappears under either two inches of rainwater or three inches of snow.

If it's snow, the hockey season is ready to start. Otherwise, dig out your basketball sneakers which should be in the back of the closet there . . . no, there . . . behind the croquet set.

And baseball season? Well, it begins on the first spring day when you can see the centerfielder's ankles from home plate. If he sinks in the mud up to his knees, it's still basketball and/or hockey season.

No self respecting kid would be seen dead chucking a baseball once football season has started. That's bad form, like wearing new Levis or combing your hair. A definite social error.

There is also a very definite season for oyster stew. Happily, most people observe it without being told.

The opening bowl of oyster stew should be served in mid-October, usually after the third day of morning frost. Oh, you can eat oysters in July, OK, but only raw, fried or in Hood Canal Stew.

Oyster stew is served normally on football Fridays. My schedule lists oyster stew every three weeks, and the season is usually climaxed in The Super Bowl, on New Year Day, because, lord, you have to have something to put out the fire.

Super Bowl Stew

For four, you'll need about a quart of fresh oysters. (Canned oysters make minor league stew, and I don't want to be involved.)

Glunk the oysters in a saucepan and if they are fairly husky, cut them in half, Simmer the oysters gently in their juices for about three or four minutes or until they begin to firm up.

Remove from heat and strain the juices into a second saucepan. Add four cups of strong chicken stock and set over low heat. In a small bowl, mix together four tablespoons soft butter and three tablespoons of flour. Slowly stir this mixture into the chicken-oyster liquid, to thicken. Add one teaspoon of Worcestershire sauce, a pinch of cayenne pepper and salt to taste.

Simmer for five minutes, then add the oysters. When they have begun to heat up, add one cup cream and reheat, but don't boil.

Serve steaming hot into four bowls, then melt a thin pat of butter in each. Goes great with:

Big League Biscuits

Make a batch of rolled biscuit dough, or else buy a roll of ready-to-cook biscuits in the supermarket.

Melt some butter and sprinkle grated parmesan cheese onto waxed paper.

Take each round biscuit, dip top in melted butter, then dip again in the parmesan cheese, place on a cookie sheet cheese side up and follow the regular instructions for baking.

We've been reading your cooking column," a Tacoma colleague remarked in a press box recently. "It's sort of interesting. But how cum you just print recipes for crud?"

"Well put, sir;" I remember thinking to myself.

It seems that the Tacoma writer, an otherwise enlightened and agreeable gentleman, defined "crud" to include oysters, clams and lamb kidneys. Apparently, he is not alone in his evaluation.

As a breed, sportswriters are culinary throwbacks to the Stone Age. If a dinosaur was hit by lightning during this early era, the cave dwellers enjoyed mixed grill. Otherwise, they munched grass or leaves, an earlier equivalent of cold breakfast food.

A sportswriter's duties often take him the length and breadth of the country. Yet the minute he arrives in New Orleans or Philadelphia or Dallas he grabs the nearest bellboy and whispers:

"Where can a guy get a good steak in this town?"

Good grief. You can get a helluva steak at the Legion Club in Cut Bank, Montana. A drunken cowboy can sear a piece of beef, if he happens to fall in the general direction of the cook wagon stove.

Give the average sportswriter a medium rare steak and a baked potato in foil and he'll happily retire to his room with a cookie. And on his travels around the country, a basketball, baseball, football or hockey writer will blithely ignore gulf prawns in New Orleans, pompano in Miami, lobster in Boston and Dungeness crab in Seattle.

Give him his choice and he'd sooner munch a hockey puck, if you call it the steak special.

The perfect way to enjoy Dungeness crab in Seattle, of course, is cold, cracked, with maybe some homemade mayonnaise or melted lemon butter on the side.

But there is a cold-weather alternate which warms and enhances the crab without overpowering it with some glucky sauce.

Cold Weather Crab

You'll need one-half of a medium-sized crab for each serving.

Clean, break the legs off the body, and quarter the main section of the crab. Crack the legs and remove large sections of the shell, so that the meat will be easy to dig out later with your crab fork. (If you have to wrestle with a hot crab leg, you'll find yourself muttering "damn" a lot.)

Place half a crab in each individual, ovenproof casserole or soup plate. Then make the following sauce:

2 cups beef bouillon
3 T. catsup
2 minced cloves garlic
1 T. soy sauce
1 T. worcestershire
2 tea. paprika

Sauce should be simmered a few minutes, then poured atop the crab. Place casseroles in 375 oven for about 20 minutes, basting frequently.

Serve with garlic bread, or this homemade alternative:

Cheese Ring

Heat a cup of milk and 1/4 cup butter in a large saucepan and add 1/2 tea. salt and a grinding of pepper. Bring to a full boil, then dump in one cup of unsifted flour. Stir over medium heat about two minutes, or until the dough forms a ball in the pan.

Remove from heat and beat in by hand, one at a time, four eggs, until the dough is once again smooth.

Grate one cup of Swiss cheese. Beat half a cup into the dough and reserve the rest.

Grease a baking sheet. Using an ice cream scoop, make seven equal-sized mounds of dough in a circle, each ball just touching the next one. Use up the remaining dough by placing a small scoop atop each large scoop. Sprinkle the remainder of the cheese over the ring and bake in center shelf of a 375 oven for 55 minutes.

The cheese ring can be removed to cool at the same time the crab is shoved into the 375 oven.

And invite some friends from Tacoma.

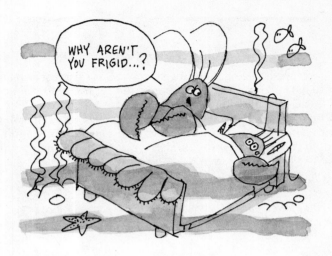

A field trip to the concrete canyons of New York a few years ago proved to at least one West Coast observer that Dungeness crab, and George Foreman's left hook, are indeed superior to Maine lobster, and Boone Kirkman's chin.

Research on Foreman and Kirkman was conducted in a Madison Square Garden ring and lasted only three minutes and 40 seconds.

That was the approximate track record for a pre-fight lobster, which was served up in a Manhattan seafood shoppe, with melted butter. Not bad, but nothing to strike terror in the heart of Ivar Haglund.

The only lobsters available fresh in Seattle arrive here on a first-class jet ticket, swim grandly around in restaurant and supermarket tanks, and cost approximately $1,000. Some additional research conducted by this department substantiated that lobsters cannot be harvested as a cash crop in the Northwest because our water isn't sexy enough. Lobsters mature sexually only in near-freezing water, like Cape Cod. The temperature in Puget Sound seldom drops below 42.

But there is really no good reason to sulk about our sexual inadequacies. Because, as we noted before, a Maine lobster would finish third in a two-way race with a Dungeness crab. The reason it would finish third is that artichokes come in second.

So why not serve up a cold supper of Dungeness crab and artichokes, on the next hot, dry day. (Research indicated that there was a hot, dry day in Seattle back in 1923.)

Certainly you don't have to be told how to clean and crack a crab. But you may be foggy on artichokes, and so:

Artichokes

Wash the artichokes and cut off the top, tough part of the stems. Attacking from the other end, next cut off the top third of the artichoke. If any thorns remain clip them off with scissors before they prompt you to cuss.

Stand the artichokes upright in a snug pan and pour a bit of white wine or lemon juice over the cut part. Pour in boiling water to cover and add one teaspoon salt. Cover and cook 40 minutes, drain and cool.

When the bell sounds for round one, alternately attack the cold crab and artichoke. The same dip can be used for both.

Crab-Artichoke Mayonnaise

Break an egg into the jar of your blender. Turn to high for 30 seconds. Add 1/2 teaspoon dry mustard, one tablespoon lemon juice and two cloves of garlic, which have been mashed in 1/2 teaspoon of salt. Add four anchovy fillets. Blend 15 seconds at high.

Pour some olive or peanut oil in a measuring cup. Turn blender to high and pour oil in thin, very slow stream. The mayonnaise will usually reach the right consistency after you have used 2/3 of the cup of oil. In any event, don't use more than a cup of oil.

The leftover mayonnaise, the remaining anchovies and some lettuce become tomorrow's salad.

If you don't like anchovy mayonnaise, and are going to be a sorehead about it, serve the crab and artichokes with one-half cup melted butter mixed with 1/2 teaspoon of dry mustard and a dash of tobasco.

Better yet, serve both dips, with garlic bread and a cup of suds, as sort of a one-two punch — for heavyweights.

Well, where do YOU stand, sir (M'am)?

Would you like to be an Oscar Mayer wiener? Do you aspire to have your children become Oscar Mayer wieners? Would you care to have an Oscar Mayer wiener move in next door to you? Can you guess what it might do to the value of your property, if the neighborhood became saturated with sausages?

These are just some of the questions being asked by the deep-thinkers of our society in this introspective era of personal consumption.

Like Nellie Shriver.

A coordinator for the American Vegetarian Association, she is waging a campaign to remove the Oscar Mayer jingle from radio commercials, and the last time we checked she had a death grip on the J. Walter Thompson Advertising Agency.

"It is our feeling that no one actually wants to be an Oscar Mayer wiener," she has explained. "We said that we felt the ad made a mockery of the intense suffering that accompanies the killing of pigs. The ad, after all, implies that something very beautiful is going to happen to pigs. The J. Walter Thompson people explained to us that it was not sung by pigs, but by children. That doesn't help"

Right on! And chances are that if the question were posed to the children on a SECRET ballot, they would disclose that they would much rather be a Hostess Twinkie, or possibly a frozen Snicker.

Let's have a little truth in advertising. And don't let Charlie the Tuna off the hook.

Nellie Shriver has no such intention. She concluded that Charlie the Tuna has definite suicidal tendencies, and she sees nothing funny about this.

Neither does talk show host Johnny Carson, who was once asked whether he thought Charlie the Tuna was mentally ill.

"I don't know," he responded. "But I think anybody who tries to psychoanalyze a fictional fish is a little weird."

Personally, I prefer to think that tunafish swim around the ocean in convenient 7-1/2 ounce cans, and are harvested by singing dolphins, just so that I can build an occasional tunafish san'ich. If the dolphins deposit two cans in your cupboard, you can serve six with the following hot dish:

Certainly, Charlie

3 T. minced onion
2 T. flour
1 T. lemon juice
1 tea. Worcestershire
dash pepper
2 shakes cayenne
2 cans tuna
4 T. margarine
3/4 cup milk
1/2 tea. dry mustard
1/2 tea. salt
1/2 tea. sage
1 egg
1/4 cup dry bread crumbs

Saute the onion in three tablespoons of the margarine, until translucent. Stir in the flour. Add milk in thin stream, stirring. Add lemon juice and remaining seasonings. When sauce is thick and hot, beat the egg in a small bowl, pour in a bit of the hot sauce, stir, then pour egg mixture back into the saucepan, stirring.

Add the tuna, heat, and spoon into six greased, individual dishes.

Mix the remaining one tablespoon of margarine with the bread crumbs and sprinkle over the top.

Bake for 20 minutes in a 350 oven.

You'll notice when you serve this dish that it still tastes like tuna fish.

Maybe you expected a filet mignon to hang itself on your fish hook?

Seagoing Spaghetti

Heat two tablespoons olive oil in a saucepan. Add 1/2 cup minced onion and one smashed clove garlic and cook until soft. Add two cans of tomato sauce and one teaspoon basil and simmer until thickened.

Add two cans flaked tuna, one can minced ripe olives, two tablespoons of capers, four anchovy fillets, salt and pepper to taste. Simmer slowly while you cook a pound of spaghetti in boiling salted water.

Drain the spaghetti when just tender, flip it onto a platter, top with the sauce. And if you don't own an authentic wineskin, you can serve the spaghetti with some chianti, out of an old hot-water bottle.

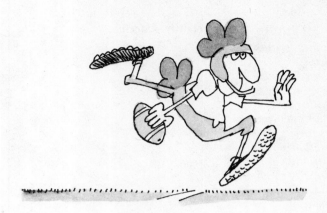

I don't want to be an alarmist, but the subject probably deserves some attention.

A usually unreliable source informs me that the high cost of meat has done more to advance the women's lib movement than Gloria Steinem. The logic is well-nigh irrefutable.

If you can't afford meat, you eat more chicken.

The more chicken you eat, the more female hormones you imbibe, due to modern poultry-raising practices designed to develop bosomy birds.

And with everybody walking around filled to the brim with female hormones . . . well, you can see that the outlook for our society is pretty alarming.

Not that an occasional drumstick is going to compel you to take up needlepoint. But you wouldn't want to bet on the Huskies against USC in football, if chicken fricassee regularly replaces blood-rare steaks at the training table. Female hormones aside, this just makes good sense. Football teams are named things like Packers, Longhorns and Bulls. "Stomp-'em, Chickens!" lacks something as a battle cry. But we digress.

What are the alternatives, with beef as precious as old gold. Macaroni and cheese and a tuna casserole? Please! Those aren't really alternatives at all.

A resident of the Pacific Northwest should consider fish. I don't think you have to worry about the hormones of anything that lays its eggs under rocks and gets them fertilized two weeks later.

You don't like fish? Well, then keep doing things to it in the pan until it doesn't taste all that much like fish.

Unfishy Fish

1 lb. fish fillets
2 chopped onions
1 T. soy sauce
salt
lemon juice
2 cloves garlic
1/2 tea. brown sugar
pepper

Rub the fillets with lemon juice. Brown lightly on each side in hot oil, reduce heat and toss in the chopped onions and the smashed garlic cloves. Fry five minutes. Mix the soy sauce with two tablespoons hot water, the sugar, some salt and pepper and a little more lemon juice. Pour over the fish, heat to boiling and serve, maybe with some potato pancakes on the side.

Blender Pancakes

Peel and cube four potatoes. Toss half the cubes into a blender, cover with ice water and whirl briefly, until potatoes are grated.

Drain the potatoes, put in a bowl, repeat process with the rest of the potatoes.

Toss into the blender two eggs (no, no, not the shells, too!) Add one chopped onion. Whirl again. Stir the egg-onion mixture in with the potatoes, add salt, pepper and as much flour as needed to slightly thicken the batter.

Fry tablespoon-sized gloops on each side in hot oil, until golden brown on both sides, drain and serve. With the fish.

P.S. According to the late bulletin from the chicken farmers, the average plucked clucker contains no more artificial female hormones than a toy truck, which is a good thing, since the next chapter is devoted to the bosomy birds.

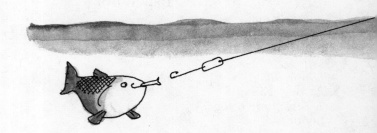

It's a wonder anybody has the stomach to eat a salmon, once it's finally hauled over the side of a boat. A charter fishing trip is not the perfect prelude to gourmet dining.

To begin with, somebody has apparently figured out that salmon eat breakfast at 6:02 a.m. Maybe so, maybe not. There's also a good chance they might sleep in until 9:15 or so if the powerboats would quit churning up the water.

But suppose they actually want to eat breakfast at 6:02? Who says you've got to take orders from a fish? Suppose your parrot decides it wants a cracker at 5:15 each morning? You going to set the alarm so he doesn't get irritated?

Yet fishermen think nothing of setting an alarm clock to feed herring to a salmon. They pour down some scalding coffee and a couple of Dramamine tablets, and go beetling out past the breakwater, headed for the whitecaps.

The next few hours are spent on the tilting deck of a bouncing boat, staring down at undulating green water, a pastime guaranteed to make the stomach fall out of Captain Ahab.

By 6 o'clock that evening the average fisherman, even the successful one, is red-eyed, irritable, and still trying to attach a mental anchor to the earth's crust. And if he has a salmon in his hand he's liable to throw it at the cat and collapse into a chair with an old chicken wing and a brownie.

Of course if you purchased a slab of salmon, or hooked your own at a civilized hour, you have the foundation for a feast. All you need is a jug of cider to create some:

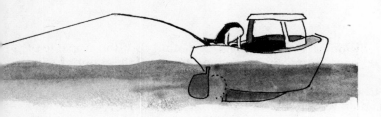

Apple Jack Salmon

Cut the salmon into steaks. Yeah, I know there's a big bone running down the middle. But you must be able to cut it into steaks. The guy at the fish market manages. Maybe there is a zipper or a snap you overlooked.

Spread both sides of the salmon steaks with prepared mustard.

Melt a quarter of a cup of butter in a skillet and add, oh, maybe a quarter of a cup of apple cider. When this ambrosia is burbling nicely, add the salmon steaks. On a 300-degree electric frying pan (or in an iron skillet over a medium bonfire) you'll want to cook the steaks about 12 minutes, then turn and cook the other side for 12 minutes, adding more cider to the pan as it bubbles away. Or, if you prefer an outdoor barbecue:

Seattle Salmon BBQ

Fillet a four-pound silver salmon, or ask your fish man to do your dirty work for you.

Sprinkle the meat side of the salmon with Accent, fresh ground pepper and authentic Indian garlic salt.

Cook skin side up at a distant setting over a hot barbecue fire for seven minutes. Turn and cook another 10 to 15 minutes. During this latter stage baste the fish with a sauce consisting of one cube melted butter, a tablespoon of Worcestershire sauce, pepper, onion salt and lots of chopped parsley.

Check the salmon with a fork and when it flakes easily load up your plate before your guests get a whiff of it.

Scientific study indicates that a single, 21-pound codfish is capable of laying 2,700,000 eggs during one spawning period. Talk about chasing around!

According to my World Book, if all the offspring of one female cod survived, you could walk from Seattle to Yokohama on a sea of cod, and that might be a bit grim on a warm day. But they don't all survive. Codfish eggs float, get eaten by the creatures of the deep, and you still have to take a boat or plane to Yokohama.

You already know more than you want to learn about codfish, but you'd still better pay attention. Because the survivors are a lot cheaper than prime rib. From the price of the latter, you can assume that virtually all of the prime rib eggs perish short of maturity.

Further study indicates that codfish dine on lobsters, shrimp and crab, although in a pinch they will settle for old scissors, spoons and rocks. In other words they just like to eat. They consider 4-1/2 pounds of seaweed sufficient as a tossed salad, but what's for dinner? So far, however, there is no evidence that they will attack man for food.

However, the reverse is not true. And the best way to attack fresh codfish is with some melted butter and a fork.

Two pounds of True Cod fillets will serve four generously, but first they need a little help. Melt a cube of butter in a saucepan. Add a half cup of olive oil, three tablespoons of vinegar, one teaspoon dry mustard, one teaspoon salt, one-half teaspoon lemon juice, one-half teaspoon savory, a minced clove of garlic and a few drops of Tabasco.

While the above ingredients simmer at low heat a few minutes, pat the fillets dry with a paper towel and toss into a shallow oven dish just big enough to hold all the fish without overlapping.

Pour the mess in the saucepan over the fillets and broil in the oven, as close as possible to the source of heat. Eight minutes should be about right, but check after five minutes and if the thickest meat is firm, white and flakes easily it's ready to eat.

This is a good way to prepare any similar fish fillets or steaks, like halibut or sole or whatever's fresh and cheap and lays 2,700,0,000 eggs.

Poultry and Game

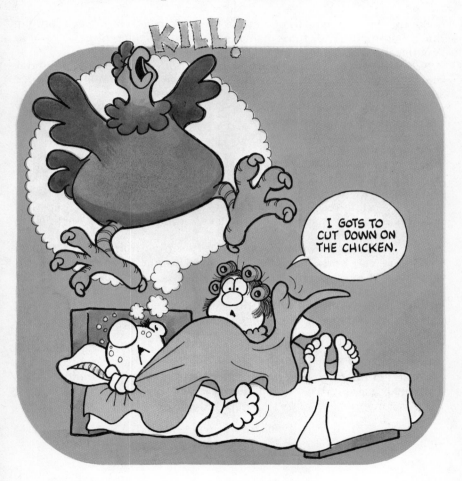

But there is one thing to be said for the people who have been running our government. They have managed to put a chicken into every pot in America. Because everything else costs $3.99 a pound.

Not that Chicken Little doesn't make a perfectly acceptable Sunday dinner. But Monday, Tuesday and Wednesday, too? Frankly, the price spiral is taxing the ingenuity of the American chef.

An associate named Phil Taylor, an avid golfer but otherwise outwardly normal, recently cooked chicken in Coca Cola and lived to tell about it. I suspect the flavor probably surpassed a Spalding Top Flite, but might fall short of a Titlist 3.

Another acquaintance swears that the only way to cook a fryer is to coat all the parts in mayonnaise, roll them in crushed cheese Ritz crackers and bake on a broiler pan in a 375 oven for an hour.

He swears the resultant dish tastes exactly like chicken coated with mayonnaise and rolled in cheese cracker crumbs, and I am inclined to believe him.

Some chicken-chasers have evolved their own homemade brand of Shake-and-You-Know-It, mixing one cup of Bisquick with two teaspoons salt, two teaspoons paprika and one teaspoon poultry seasoning. You can store it in a glass jar and, when ready to attack the poultry, shake the chicken pieces in a sack full of the mixture. Melt 1/2 cup margarine in baking dish, add the chicken pieces skin side down and bake 45 minutes at 350. Turn, bake 15 minutes more, and serve.

The following recipe is a trifle more complicated, but involves no expensive ingredients except for the chicken, which admittedly has increased in price the past few frantic years. But it's still running a poor third behind a rump roast and a jumbo prawn, so grab one by the leg as it goes past if you'd like to try the following recipe.

Undressed Chicken

1 fryer
salt, pepper
2 eggs
lard
1 lemon
flour
bread crumbs
half cube margarine

Cut the chicken into serving pieces and remove the skin from all the pieces except the wings. (If you try to undress the wings you're going to be standing there until Thursday, and I'm getting hungry.)

Remove some of the bones from the two breast pieces, so they'll lie flat.

Cut the lemon in half and squeeze some juice over both sides of the chicken pieces. Let it sit at room temperature for about an hour.

Pat chicken dry with paper towel, sprinkle both sides with salt and pepper and coat lightly with flour.

Mix the two beaten eggs with two tablespoons of water. Dip each chicken piece into the egg mixture, roll in the bread crumbs and then let it sit on that waxed paper over there for about 20 minutes, so the glue will dry.

You want the lard in your skillet almost half an inch deep, which should use up a little over half a pound. The fat shouldn't be at top heat, but when it begins to undulate seductively around the pan it's time to add the chicken.

Cook until golden, about six minutes on each side. Reduce heat and cook another six minutes on each side. Meanwhile melt the margarine.

Remove the chicken to an oven platter, pour some margarine over each piece, let it bake 10 minutes at 350 and serve, maybe with:

New Potatoes

Scrape enough potatoes for four, cut in quarters and toss into a pot. Add one teaspoon salt, 1/2 teaspoon sugar and boiling water to barely cover.

Cook uncovered five minutes. Cover and cook another 10-12 minutes, until just tender. Pour off the water, shake pan over low heat for a minute, then plunk in three tablespoons butter. Cook, stirring a couple of times, until the potatoes are golden. You can toss some cooked (not canned) green peas in with them. Course, you could also cook the chicken in Coke. Takes all kinds . . .

63

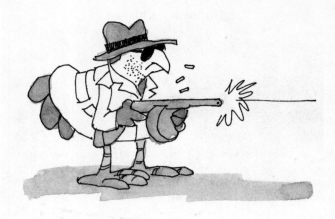

Godfather Chicken

Cut the chicken into serving pieces, wash, and pat dry. Rub the pieces with salt and pepper. Then dip in two beaten eggs and roll in a mixture consisting of 3/4 cup fine breadcrumbs and 3/4 cup grated parmesan cheese.

Heat 1/3 cup olive oil in heavy skillet, add the chicken and brown on all sides, turning frequently. When browned, reduce heat and fry for another 30 minutes.

If you want to get rid of the rest of that parmesan, try this as a side dish.

Baked Asparagus

Cut off the heavy ends of the asparagus and arrange in a skillet. Pour in boiling water to cover and add 1/2 teaspoon of salt. Bring to a boil and cook uncovered for five minutes, depending upon size of asparagus spears.

Remove spears from the skillet and arrange in a baking dish. Top with a mixture consisting of 1/3 cup melted butter and half a cup of dry, white wine. Sprinkle with salt, pepper and grated parmesan cheese, shove into a 425 oven and serve after 10 minutes. What, you've STILL got a hole in your stomach?

Grate Potatoes

Peel and coarsely grate (get it?) eight potatoes. Add one tablespoon grated onion, three beaten eggs, a cup of scalded milk, 1/3 cup of butter and a teaspoon salt. Mix together in greased dish and bake an hour at 250.

Curried Chicken

Dismember a fryer and wipe dry. In a paper bag dump a cup of Bisquick, two tablespoons of curry powder (or less, if you think small), one-half tablespoon of salt and one-quarter teaspoon pepper.

Shake the chicken, a couple of pieces at a time, in this mixture until coated, and set aside.

Preheat your oven to 425 and meanwhile pour a quarter-cup of shortening and a quarter-cup of butter into a large Pyrex oven pan (or whatever). Put it into the heated oven until the shortening begins to sputter, then quickly add the chicken (skin side down) and bake for 40 minutes.

Reduce the temperature to 375 degrees, turn the chicken, cook 20 minutes more and serve.

The first time I attempted this, I coated the chicken in a plastic bag which I cleverly set down on the opened oven door while tossing the chicken into the pan.

The plastic melted, the curried flour poured out onto the hot oven door, was swept in panic onto the kitchen floor which soon — with the assistance of a mop and a sprinkling of water — resembled the bed of the Ganges River during a severe drought.

But the chicken tasted great, if you watched where you walked.

Potato Balls

Peel some baking spuds, then scoop out rounds of potatoes with a melon ball cutter. Parboil the balls in slightly salted water for three minutes, then drain.

Melt lotsa butter in the frying pan, toss in the potato balls and fry lightly, shaking the pan occasionally, until the balls have a golden crust. Sprinkle with salt and parsley and serve.

65

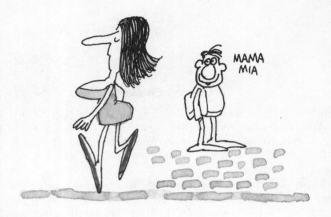

Granted, some people are offended by padded breasts, but you have to respect their . . . errr . . . views.

"How can you improve upon nature?" they argue.

And there is a basic flaw in confusing biggest with best, although you'll never convince some Italians.

Italy seems to be the center for the bountiful bosom philosophy, and the explanation is twofold.

Prosciutto . . .

And mozzarella.

A chicken breast wrapped around a little prosciutto and melted mozzarella is . . . well, "voluptuous" is probably the only way to describe it.

Genuine Italian Breasts entail a little effort and a modest investment. But what makes it all worthwhile is that you are going to have some prosciutto left over, and do I have a lunch for you tomorrow!

Have your Italian grocer carve up a half pound of the smoked ham in paper thin slices. As I say, you really don't need a half pound, but buy it anyway. You can't interrupt a busy Italian grocer and tell him you want one-sixteenth of a pound of prosciutto, two chi chi beans and three strands of spaghetti.

Busy Italian grocers have got a lot more to do than, say, busy Irish grocers. They've got to construct 3,217 raviolis, stuff a half-mile of sausage casings, grate 83 pounds of parmesan cheese, milk a goat, write a thank-you letter to Marlon Brando and be finished before early Mass.   ·

So buy the half pound, and a fist-sized hunk of mozzarella to construct:

Genuine Italian Breasts

To amply serve four guests, buy four chicken breasts, skin, bone and halve them, place each one between two slices of waxed paper and whack lustily with the flat side of a heavy butcher knife, until they are flattened and almost doubled in diameter.

Sprinkle each flattened breast with salt and pepper, top with two slices of prosciutto, some grated mozerella and roll up to completely enclose the stuffing. If you have a tidy mind, go ahead and shove a toothpick through each breast so that it won't come unglued.

Dust the breasts with seasoned flour. Heat 1/4 cup olive oil over medium heat in a skillet and brown breasts on all sides. Remove to a baking dish.

Pour off oil but retain the brown nummies in the pan. Add one cup dry white wine to the skillet and boil for one minute, scraping bottom of pan with a wooden spoon. Add two cups of tomato sauce, two teaspoons of oregano, salt and pepper. Pour over breasts and bake in 350 oven, for 15 minutes. Sprinkle with parsley and serve, maybe with some cooked seashell macaroni.

See, you have plenty of prosciutto left over for tomorrow's lunch, which happens to be a modest, no-cal repast known as:

Fatman's Fettuccine

To amply serve three (somebody must have dropped out by now) you'll need about one-half pound fettuccini noodles, half a cup of shredded prosciutto, half a cup of grated parmesan cheese, half a cup of fresh or frozen peas which have been cooked until just tender, 1/4 cup of warm cream and 1/4 cup butter, cut into pieces.

Cook the fettuccine noodles in salted boiling water until done (about eight minutes). Meanwhile toss the pieces of butter into a large serving dish and place in a just-warm oven.

Drain the fettuccine quickly in a collander, dump it into the serving dish, toss until it is all covered with butter, add the parmesan, cream, peas and ham, continue to toss until thoroughly mixed, and serve at once on hot plates.

If that hasn't stuffed your breast, there just might be enough scraps of cheese and ham left over for a poorboy sandwich.

I don't know whether it is being produced by Weyerhaeuser or the Simpson Timber Co., but somebody has come out with this sensational wood byproduct which could solve the world's food problems.

Just think, breaded veal cutlets, mass produced, machine stamped and flash frozen, without any veal, and precious little bread.

One report has it that the research scientists were attempting to develop a new acoustical tile and were inspecting various samples during a company lunch, when one accidentally fell in the mashed potatoes.

"Say!" an ambitious junior vice president exclaimed. "With a little gravy on this, it almost looks like a breaded veal cutlet."

Three months later, enhanced by onion flakes (actually seasoned pine chips) and parsley (reclaimed swamp moss), New Products Division declared the ersatz veal cutlets ready for the market.

And it really is a marvelous product, and a boon to the busy housewife and/or prison chef. Grilled carefully, according to precise instructions, the cutlet tastes exactly like acoustical wallboard which has fallen into somebody's mashed potatoes and gravy.

But do you know something awful? An entire generation is being raised under the misapprehension that THIS is Veal!

And it isn't!

Veal is actually the flesh of young calves with big eyes and . . . well, never mind about that.

Thin, tender slices of veal, sauteed slowly with fine cheeses and wines, repose at the very foundation of fine Italian cuisine.

Unfortunately, thin, tender slices of Real Veal currently are more expensive than an unfortunate marriage. And your tongue is going to fall out onto the sidewalk if you as much as suggest that Sooper-Serve has a special on flash-frozen wallboard.

Better you should construct something which could be called:

Unreal Veal

One chicken breast will handsomely serve each eater. Remove the skin, cut and claw and swear a little until you have separated the meat from the bone and gristle. Now you have two nice fillets of chicken from each breast, right?

Flatten by placing the chicken between two pieces of waxed paper, and then driving a Chevvy half-ton over the top. (Or you can pound it with a rolling pin or wine bottle, if you're low on gas.)

Place a three-inch by quarter-inch, by quarter-inch piece of Monterrey Jack cheese inside each flattened, salted and peppered breast, roll and fold the meat into a neat packet and secure with a toothpick.

Mix an egg with two tablespoons of water. Dip the chicken packet into the mixture, roll in bread crumbs and place in an oven dish.

Combine a can of mushroom soup with one cup of milk and two tablespoons of sherry. Surround, but do not cover, the chicken with this mixture.

Cover with foil and cook one hour at 350 degrees. Uncover, cook another 15 minutes, and serve, maybe with a side dish of:

Herbed Cauliflower

Wash a head of you-know-what and remove any brown spots (or green ones, for that matter). Drop Cauliflower into a deep pan which contains three inches of boiling, salted water. Cover, cook 15 to 20 minutes until just tender.

Drain, remove to a warm dish.

Melt a stick of butter or Mother-Nature-Fooler. Toss in two tablespoons minced parsley, one tablespoon of minced green onion tops, a tablespoon of lemon juice and one teaspoon of dried thyme.

Pour this over the top of the cauliflower and serve.

You say you need something green on the plate to go with the white chicken and the white cauliflower. OK, double the amount of parsley. Or, better yet, substitute some reconstituted swamp moss.

If a guy were casting a vote for Comeback of the Year, he'd have to give some serious consideration to the soybean.

Health fadists are substituting soy chops for sirloin. Cows, pigs and goats are running wind sprints across the barnyard towards the feed bin, when soybeans are on the menu. Suddenly, Iowa farmers are planting all their acreage in soybeans and are financing fabulous vacation villas in Dubuque, with the profits.

You have to admit that constitutes a heckuva rally, for a commodity once deemed fit only for the manufacture of bug juice.

For the first 12 years of my life, I thought soy sauce actually was bug juice. The family would frequently visit a favorite Chinese restaurant, my father would invariably order a bowl of noodles and a side order of barbecued pork, and while he was waiting for the waiter to bring it, he would ceremoniously hoist his soup spoon, fill it from the black bottle on the table, and suck it down raw.

"Bug juice!" my sister and I would croak, and fall heavily to the floor, cross-eyed, clutching our throats.

I don't know who first told us it was bug juice. Probably my father. And anything served in a black bottle and which obviously could not be identified as catsup was suspect.

Soy beans' reputation was not enhanced by World War II. Suddenly, all the O'Henrys, Babe Ruths and frozen Snickers began to disappear from the corner grocery store, to be replaced by five-cent sacks of salted soybeans.

They were not an adequate substitute, for at least three reasons. It was difficult to eat enough so that you could properly spoil your dinner, they were noticeably ineffective at creating cavities, and they wouldn't even melt in your pants pocket. So much for salted soybeans. We gutted it out until the armistice, and a resulting avalanche of Mr. Goodbars.

The fact that sacks of salted soybeans almost immediately vanished with the end of the war led to the logical conclusion that the Japanese had been forced to accept them as a part of the armistice agreement. We got Okinawa and the Bonin Islands, Russia got the Southern Kuriles, and Japan was stuck with all the salted soybeans that China didn't eat.

The way China and Japan have rebounded since 1946 would indicate clearly that the soybean is a much more versatile commodity than, say, Okinawa, and the demand for both beans and bug juice is unprecedented in this country, even among the younger set.

Kids today holler and scream for soy sauce on their hamburgers teriyaki, their chicken Hawaiian, and they'd probably pour it on their Cheerios, if you let them.

Don't. Instead, serve them some:

Bug Juice Chicken

Cut a fryer into serving-size pieces and place in oven pan, skin side down.

Pour one-third cup of soy sauce into a measuring cup, add two tablespoons of lemon juice and 1/4 teaspoon each of onion powder, garlic powder, poultry seasoning and powdered ginger.

Pour the soy mixture over the chicken, flip the coated chicken skin side up and bake in a 375 oven for 75 minutes, basting twice with the pan juices.

When the chicken is almost done, cook enough noodles to serve four in boiling, salted water.

Drain noodles, remove chicken to a warm dish, then dump the noodles into the oven pan and moosh 'em around in the remaining soy mixture. Gloop the noodles — sauce and all — into a serving dish, sprinkle with minced parsley and pass them around, close behind the platter of chicken, maybe with some Chinese pea pods on the side.

And if you eat up all your chicken and noodles and peas, you can have a frozen Snicker for dessert.

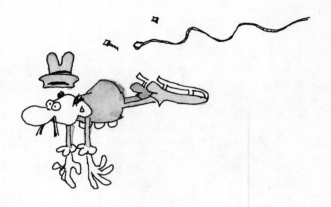

Freddie Trenkler is an ice skating clown who frequently performed in Seattle and the climax of his act called for him to soar grandly above the spectators on a wire, connected to the ceiling of the Coliseum.

He performed this stunt several years ago on the Ed Sullivan TV Show. But on that particular occasion it was more of a sore than a soar. Because Freddie Trenkler, pixie-clown, suddenly found himself imitating Clarence the Cannonball, as the result of an equipment malfunction.

"Thank yew vedy much, Freddie Trenkler," I believe Sullivan ended that particular show. "Be sure to tune in next week, on our show, when we will present a collision between a Datsun and the Empire Builder . . . "

"Equipment malfunction" is an euphemism for "I thought YOU, tightened the bolt," and that was one explanation for the accident. Some of Freddie's friends have an alternate theory.

A Vienna native and an avid amateur chef, Trenkler would sometimes shove a succulent roast into a slow oven, race to the arena, perform his pratfalls, and return to his motel or apartment in time to mash the potatoes.

It's just possible that at the apex of his swing, he recalled that the recipe specified 40 minutes a pound in a 300 oven instead of 30 minutes a pound in a 400 oven. If true, his hasty departure was fully justified.

And there could be even a third explanation. Trenkler's French wife, Gigi, would sometimes accompany him on tour. And he'd probably beetle back to the motel after each performance even if she were parboiling some of his old ice skate liners. Instead, she probably was cooking up some:

72

Vienna Chicken Paprika

5 slices bacon
4 T. paprika
2 chicken bouillon cubes
2 T. wine vinegar
1 T. sour cream
1 chicken
1 T. flour
1 diced onion
1 tea. salt
pepper

In a heavy skillet cook the diced bacon slowly until medium done. Remove bacon bits from pan and toss in the diced onion. When it begins to brown remove, turn up the heat, and brown the chicken pieces until golden brown on all sides.

Fling the onion and bacon back into the pan atop the chicken, sprinkle with the vinegar, paprika, salt and a generous grinding of pepper. Dissolve the bouillon cubes in four cups of hot water and add to the pan.

Cover and cook slowly for 30 minutes. Remove chicken to a warm dish in the oven. Mix the flour with a small amount of water and two tablespoons of the sludge now gurgling in the pan. Stir the flour mixture back into the pan and cook mixture until it begins to thicken.

Remove pan from heat for 27.345 seconds (or approximately half a minute), then stir in the sour cream, reheat to a simmer and pour the sauce over the cooked chicken. The cream shouldn't curdle since you let the mixture cool but if it does, swear a little and beat it with a wire whip.

Gigi Trenkler said that in Vienna, this dish is served atop rice with white wine or beer, a tossed salad, and a pastry or a carmel pudding.

In Seattle it's served atop cooked and salted noodles with a side dish of broccoli in hollandaise sauce and a slab of cheese cake and no wonder the wire broke!

Kareem Jabbar is paid a zillion dollars a year to dunk a basketball in Milwaukee, Derek Sanderson once received $1 million not to play hockey in Philadelphia, and your average saddle bronc rider is on the shorts.

Measured against other professional athletes, the rodeo performer is drastically underpaid. The amateurs earn even less.

You should understand at the beginning that when Jim Plunkett plays the Lions, he actually only has to contend with some overweight gentlemen from Detroit, who growl a lot. However, when Larry Mahan plays the Bulls, he is playing real bulls, equipped with all the standard equipment like horns, overdrive and power steering.

When Jack Nicklaus hits a golf ball, he is usually pretty certain it won't hit him back. Ace Berry is protected by no written or unwritten guarantee, when he yells Yahoooo at a mount known as Descent.

I might suggest that rodeo riders go on strike, except that would mean they would have to return home to communities like Burkburnett, Texas, and Sedan, Kansas. An occasional kick in the head is probably preferable to a weekend in Hugo, Oklahoma.

Another legitimate complaint concerns the food cowboys are forced to eat. Suppose you were going to invite some calf-ropers over to your house for an evening of arm wrestling. What would you serve them? Barbecued beef and beans, right?

Did it ever occur to you they are probably having barbecued beef and beans shoved at them 163 days a year? The obvious reason cowboys walk so funny is that they are full of beans.

Barbara Rutherford has come up with a viable alternative. Wife of a rodeo official, she obviously feeds a lot of hungry steer-punchers, and an occasional sickly sheepherder. Know what she feeds them? Clucking cattle, alias chicken. But she prepares it in a hot buffet dish which she calls:

Viva la Chicken Casserole

3 or 4 whole chicken breasts
1 dozen corn tortillas
1 can cream of chicken soup (undiluted)
1 can cream of mushroom soup (undiluted)
1 cup milk
1 grated onion
two 4-ounce cans green chili sauce (salsa)
1 lb. grated cheddar cheese (or maybe a little bit less)

Cook the chicken in simmering water to cover or wrap in foil and bake one hour at 350. Butter a large, shallow baking dish. If you cooked the chicken in foil pour any juices into the baking dish, too.

Remove skin and bones from the cooked breasts, break the chicken up into big hunks. Cut tortillas (thawed, if you bought them frozen) into one-inch-wide strips.

Mix the soup with the milk, onion and chili sauce.

Place a layer of tortilla strips in the bottom of the baking dish. Scatter some chicken hunks over the tortillas, spoon some of the sauce over the chicken, and then build up more layers of tortillas, chicken and sauce until you've used up all the ingredients.

Scatter the grated cheese over the top and toss in a 350 oven for one hour.

Mrs. Rutherford suggests letting the layered casserole sit in the refrigerator for 24 hours before cooking it, to give the flavors a chance to blend. We found that's an 'excellent idea, unless your guests look like they're getting restless after eight or nine hours.

P.S. It'll serve approximately seven cowboys or 10 sheepherders.

"People told us it was impossible to put on a World's Fair on 75 acres of land in a crowded section of the city," former mayor Dorm Braman reminisced a couple of years back. "We were urged to buy a thousand acres at Midway, and move the fair out there. Well, if we had, that's what we'd have today — a meadow in Midway, not what we have at the Seattle Center."

What we have at the Seattle Center today is grass, trees, flowers, music, some wild fountains and soaring white columns. We also used to have a lot of scruffy teen-agers who inquired, "Can I please have your change, mister?"

But the Seattle Center management won its running battle with scruffy teenagers. In the event one left his favorite plot of grass in search of a comfort station, the Seattle Center staff would immediately rush out with a shovel, plant a geranium on the spot, and erect a sign reading:

NEW PLANTING . . . PLEASE KEEP OFF

And how can you get mad at a geranium?

The Seattle Center has a science pavilion and an art gallery and a fun forest with a ride which satisfactorily shakes everybody's teeth out in 13-1/2 seconds.

You can gamble at the Seattle Center, tossing baseballs at milk bottles and throwing darts at balloons but a few years ago John Law raided the plastic ducks, with the lucky numbers on the bottom, because it looked too much like a floating crap game.

Oh yea, the Seattle Center also has FOOD, in season.

You can invest in a meatball sandwich, fish and chips, an egg roll and rice or a Mongolian steak at the Food Circus.

A typical three-course meal consists of a pizza slice, a pronto pup and a slab of lemon meringue pie. Nutritious, satisfying and slenderizing (provided you specify no-cal pizza and pie.)

A personal favorite was the barbecued chicken once served at a corner rib pit. The following recipe approaches this feast, so let's call it:

Food Circus Chicken

Purchase one split broiler half for each free loader. Brush with melted butter.

Place the chicken halves on oven broiler, leg side up, five inches from heat, and broil 10 minutes. Brush with melted butter, turn and broil other side 10 minutes.

Lower the pan six inches from the heat and broil, turning frequently and basting with barbecue sauce. If the chicken begins to char, lower heat to 500. It will be done in 45 minutes to an hour. And it can be held at a low oven temperature while you're throwing together the remainder of the meal, maybe a little seasoned rice and some asparagus, which they don't sell at the Food Circus.

BBQ Sauce for Baste
(For Four)

1/2 cup vinegar
1 tea. Worcestershire
split clove garlic
3/4 tea. salt
1-1/2 T. catsup
tabasco to taste
1/3 cup salad oil
1/2 tea. grated onion
1T. brown sugar
1/4 tea. paprika
1/4 tea. dry mustard
liquid smoke to taste

Mix all ingredients and simmer 15 minutes.

At the instant the chicken rounds third base and heads for home, chop the white ends off the slender, fresh asparagus, wash and place in a wide frying pan. Add water almost to cover, bring to fast boil, cover and cook 5-10 minutes, or until tender. Drain, add salt and copious butter and serve with the chicken and rice.

When was the last time you spotted a flock of roosters, flying overhead?

Not lately, I'll wager.

You see, they fly only on moonless nights. Veterans of jet travel might occasionally spot the odd flock were they not otherwise involved watching (1) the in-flight movies, (2) the stewardii or (3) the port engine, for tell-tale sparks. If you did suspect something flashed past your window on the approach to O'Hare, you're right. It was a flight of roosters.

Oh, they're sneaky about it. By day, they cluck around the barnyard looking aerodynamically unsound and trying to prove it with an occasional five-yard flight ending in an explosion of feathers and chicken-curses. By night, however, they soar into the clouds, headed for distant barnyards and foreign lovers.

The evidence of their flight is overwhelming, if second hand. For beginners, each chicken is equipped with two (2) wings, standard issue for robins, ducks and the Boeing 707. They have wings, ergo they must fly.

Beyond that chickens, and chicken wings are found in supermarkets, vendor stalls and country markets on every continent, a staple of diets in Pakistan, Peking and the Texas Panhandle. Obviously, they're moving pretty fast.

Poultry distributors are all somewhat embarrassed by this. Hardly anyone gets to see the chickens fly, but here they are trying to peddle wings. Consequently they often offer them for sale at distress prices.

They're excellent as appetizers, midnight snacks or even as the mainstay of the meal, if you like chicken wings.

Remove the tips and cut the wings at the joint so you have two small pieces from each. Marinate them for a few hours, then place on a lightly greased pan, cover loosely with aluminum foil and toss them into a 350 oven for about 25 to 30 minutes, removing foil twice to baste.

To crisp the wings, cook them another 5-10 minutes with the foil removed.

On the next page are some appropriate marinades.

Pakistan

1/4 cup olive oil
1 tea. grated lemon peel
1/4 tea. pepper
Smashed clove garlic
3 drops tabasco
1/4 cup lemon juice
1/2 tea. salt
1/2 tea. onion powder
1 tea. chili powder
3 T. catsup

(Mix and pour over chicken.)

Peking

1/3 cup soy sauce
1/2 tea. ginger
1/4 cup brown sugar
1/4 cup water
1/3 cup sherry
2 minced green onions

(Heat until sugar dissolves, pour over chicken.)

Panhandle

1/2 cup oil
1/2 cup catsup
1/4 tea. oregano
1/4 cup chopped onion
1 tea. chili powder
1/3 cup vinegar
1/2 cup fruit juice
1 tea. tabasco
2 tea. salt

(Boil two minutes, cool and pour over chicken.)
It's obvious that the Panhandle recipe will give you more marinade than the Peking recipe which will give you more than the Pakistan recipe so adjust according to your needs.

After all, how am I to know how many chickens are going to crash-land in your yard?

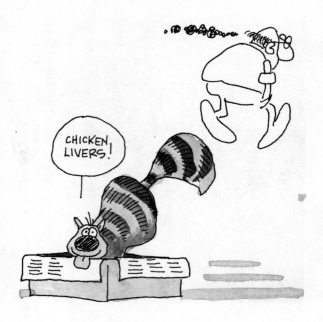

Take one pound of chicken livers . . .

Know something interesting? Eighty-four per cent of the readers who first read those instructions in The Seattle Post-Intelligencer used that page of the paper to line the cat's box.

Chicken livers . . . rip . . . cat's box. Just like that! Remarkable reaction, right?

Since the above statistic is semi-scientific, someone might conclude that an Intermediate Eater with his head screwed on straight would ignore this particular peninsula of cuisine. Not at all. The very thought shakes the basic foundations of editorial integrity and completely ignores the fact that I like chicken livers.

You don't like chicken livers? That's your weird aberration. Go print your own recipe, fella! (M'am!) What do I care? If you all liked chicken livers they'd cost $2.34 a pound and I couldn't afford them.

Besides, why should this column sink to the lowest common denominator of culinary achievement? How many recipes do you need for meat loaf and mashed 'tatters? Go drown another wiener. Try sucking on a frozen chicken pie.

The discriminating 16 per cent will dine in style.

Sherried Livers

1 lb. chicken livers
1/2 cup chicken broth
3 T. oil
2 T. soy sauce
2 T. sherry
1 T cornstarch
1/2 cup sliced onions

Cut the livers in half. Heat the oil and saute the onions until soft. Add the livers and fry, stirring occasionally, until brown on all sides. Add broth, bring to a low boil, cover and cook two minutes.

Stir the cornstarch into the sherry-soy mixture and dribble this slowly into the pan, stirring. When sauce thickens, serve over toasted English muffins or with rice.

Livers and Mushrooms

You'll need a pound of chicken livers and a half pound of fresh mushrooms. No, I'd resist that cluster of pods in the back yard. Granted, they are dirt cheap. But a factory increase in the price of stomach pumps has just been announced.

Cut the livers in half. Quarter the mushrooms. Saute the livers and mushrooms in 1/4 cup butter. When the livers are browned on the outside, stir in one tablespoon flour, 1/2 tea. salt, 1/2 tea. fine herbs, 1/2 cup chicken bouillon and 1/4 cup of dry white wine.

Simmer the livers a couple more minutes, occasionally scraping the bottom of the pan. Again, serve with rice or toasted muffins, and maybe with a big frosted glass of tomato juice which has been rendered palatable by a squirt of lemon juice, a splash of Worcestershire sauce, a zip of tabasco, flick of celery salt and a grinding of black pepper.

The supermarkets call them turkey hindquarters. Hopefully they are not the residue from some calamitous barnyard accident. Presumably the front quarters are destined for those antiseptic "turkey roasts" which will give birth to 10 million hot turkey sans, at a thousand roadside eateries.

Never mind the dashboard. We're concerned with the rumble seat, which can easily be transformed into a great, and relatively inexpensive dinner for four, with enough left over for a midnight sandwich, or two.

If you decide to barbecue, light a medium hot fire and while it is heating up melt a cube of butter (euphemism for margarine) and add a squeeze or two of lemon juice. Baste the turkey on both sides, then sprinkle liberally with a mixture comprised of two parts sugar to one part each salt and paprika, plus a grinding of pepper.

Place the turkey hindquarter on the grill, cut side down, cover with aluminum foil, and cook 45 minutes. Turn, baste again, cover again and cook for another hour. Fling the left-over salt-paprika-sugar mixture into the melted butter. Turn the turkey haunch twice during the last 15-20 minutes, basting with the butter mixture.

The dark meat will have the expensive flavor of smoked turkey, parts of the neck and wings will be charred, crisp and terrific.

However, if it rains, you can cook the turkey in a 325 oven. Baste, sprinkle, and cook skin side down for one hour. Turn, sprinkle again and cook, basting often, two more hours (or until thermometer reads 175). This won't have the smoked-turkey flavor, but is imminently satisfactory.

If you do cook this in the oven, you can toss together a potato casserole side dish faster than the 60-yard dash at the Weight Watcher's Picnic.

Cheeeeese! Potatoes

Make up enough mashed potatoes for six. You can use one of the better-brand instant mashed potatoes, because we're going to glunk some goop on it.

Mash two garlic cloves and toss into a pan. Add a can of cheese soup, two teaspoons of salt and 1/3 cup milk. Mix slowly until smooth. Put the mashed potatoes into a greased casserole. Pour the cheese mixture on top, sprinkle with buttered bread crumbs and shove it into the oven 30 minutes before the turkey is done.

Question: How do you stuff a turkey hindquarter?
Answer: You don't, but if you still demand dressing:

Pan-Cooked Dressing

While the turkey is cooking toss the gizzard and liver and the neck into a saucepan and add salted water to cover. Toss in a celery top and a peeled and quartered small onion. Simmer until gizzard is tender. Remove and chop gizzard and liver. Remove meat from neck, but reserve liquid. Assemble the following:

1 minced onion
3/4 cup parsley
1 tea. Kitchen Bouquet
1-1/2 cubes melted butter
1/4 tea. white pepper
1/2 tea. sage
1/4 tea. salt
1-1/4 cups minced celery
1/2 tea. poultry seasoning
loaf white bread

Combine the onion, chopped parsley, celery with butter and seasonings. Add 1-1/2 cups of the water from that gizzard mess on the stove. Stir in the Kitchen Bouquet. Break the bread into small pieces and toss into the bowl with the other ingredients. Mix well, and toss the whole schmeer into a large, flat oven pan.

Cover with aluminum foil and put on the shelf under the turkey quarter during the final 45 minutes of cooking time.

Sheeee, Gravy Too?

When the turkey is done remove to a hot platter. Remove rack from the pan if you used one and spoon off most of the fat, leaving only 3 tablespoons of drippings in the bottom of pan.

Stir in three tablespoons of flour, scraping up all the brown specks of succulence from bottom of pan. Pour the rest of the water from the gizzard pan into a measuring cup and add enough water from tap to make 2-1/2 cups total.

Pour the water into the pan over heat, stir up with the flour-dripping mixture and bring to a boil, continuing to stir until thickened. Add gizzard-liver-neck meat, warm with gravy, then pour into heated gravy bowl.

If you also need a cranberry fix, you're on your own.

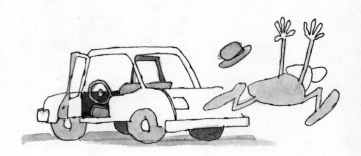

A couple residing east of the lake once phoned their 14-year-old daughter in the late afternoon, told her they'd be home in about an hour, and asked her to put the ham into a 350 oven.

Who says kids don't mind? That exactly what she did . . . put the ham into a 350 oven.

Of course, it might have been better if she had put the ham into a pan and then into a 350 oven, but actually things worked out OK. I believe her next 4-H project was an essay on:

"How to Transform an Electric Oven into a Community Smudge Pot."

I don't recall whether her mother got the oven cleaned in time for a Thanksgiving turkey, or whether they just decided to smoke another ham.

Of course, it is possible to cook turkey in a frying pan. But this shouldn't be attempted until the bird has reached the terminal stages of consumption.

There is a magic moment when the kids begin to snarl at the prospect of another hot turkey sandwich. You could belt them with some turkey soup, but by tradition the bird is not ready for the pot until:

A — At least seven ribs are showing or . . .

B — It has been rejected by the cat.

In the interim, consider turkey hash.

No, not just any turkey hash. The recipe on the next page was handed down to me by a 90-year-old New England native, who I believe clipped it out of a 1969 copy of Playboy.

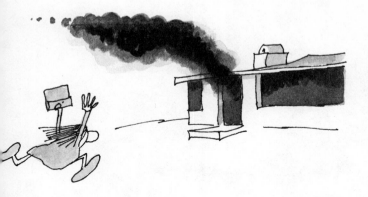

Terminal Turkey

3 cups diced leftover turkey
1/2 cup cream or milk
1/2 cup soft bread crumbs
1/2 cup chopped green pepper
2 T. chopped parsley
2 T. butter
2 T. flour
1/2 cup chopped onion
1/2 tea. salt and a grinding of pepper
1/2 tea. sage

Toss the turkey, crumbs, green pepper, onion, parsley and seasonings into a big bowl. In a saucepan melt two tablespoons of butter, blend in flour and cream and stir until thickened. Gloop this mixture into the bowl and run your fingers through everything for awhile.

Melt the remaining two tablespoons of butter in a large frying pan. When it is bubbling, toss in the turkey mixture and cook, uncovered, for 25 minutes.

Of course, you're going to have a difficult time manufacturing any turkey hash unless you first cook a turkey. Just try tossing it into a 350 oven. For beginners.

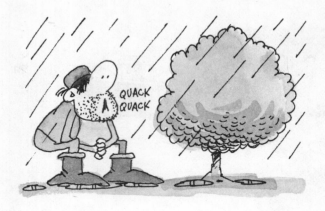

Now if this is the way you like to spend your day off, the opportunities are abundant, and you don't have to drive halfway across the state. Merely pick some particularly dismal weekend when the rain is hammering neat holes in your roof, and set your Saturday morning alarm clock for 5:15.

When it rings, run into the kitchen, grab a pitcher of ice water out of the refrigerator, pour exactly one cupful into each of your rubber boots, finish dressing, trot out into the front yard, find a comfortable spot in the garden mud and hunch down behind the rhododendron bush. Just remain that way, in an alert crouch, for the better part of the day. If you want to holler "Quack! Quack!" a couple of times, feel free, although that'll make you fair game for that Hound of the Baskervilles in the next yard.

Then in the afternoon you can wander down to Pike Place or your neighborhood supermarket, and buy a duck. Granted, it'll cost you about five bucks. But that's the cheap way to promote a duck dinner.

The alternative is to purchase a Browning Over-And-Under shotgun for about $400, a waterfowl permit and a few decoys, and drive over to Toppenish. The gas will cost you about $7, you can find a motel for $15, set aside another $7 for food, the box of shotgun shells you'll use to pollute the atmosphere is worth about $5 and don't forget to make a stop at the State Store, to pick up a $3.50 pint of mouthwash. The ducks won't come near you if they can smell your breath.

As you can see, $5 isn't a lot to pay for a duck, and it should buy about a six-pounder for a family of four.

Market Mallard

If the duck is frozen it will thaw overnight at room temperature. Remove the giblet, heart and liver, which nature has thoughtfully packaged in a little paper sack, and reserve.

Wash the duck, pat dry inside and out. Cut a lemon in half and squeeze it inside the bird. Sprinkle the bird with salt and pepper, inside and out. Rub the skin with a split clove of garlic, place duck atop a rack in a roasting pan. Prick the skin of the duck with a fork in about a dozen places, and shove bird into a 375 oven.

Roast for 30 minutes, remove duck and rack from pan briefly, pour off the fat, add one cup of dry white wine and return duck and rack to the pan. Reduce heat to 350 and cook for about 20 minutes per pound, basting with the wine. Total cooking time for our six-pound bird was about two hours and 10 minutes. By that time the skin was dark brown and crackly and the drumstick wiggled enticingly.

Remove duck to a heated platter and set it in a warm place while you continue.

Skim the fat from the pan drippings, and there'll be quite a lot. To the remaining brown drippings in the pan add one-half cup of chicken bouillon or stock, the juice of two oranges, juice of one lemon and three tablespoons of sherry.

Let all of this burble atop your stove while you mix two tablespoons of sugar in another small pan. Heat and stir until this mixture turns golden, then stir that into the pan drippings. Simmer until reduced by half. If you wish a thicker sauce mix some cornstarch with water and stir in as the sauce simmers.

Pour the sauce into a serving boat and, if you like add some thin slices of orange rind. (Peel one orange, thin enough to avoid any of the bitter, white pith. Slice and cook three minutes in boiling water.)

Carve the duck, serve portions on four heated plates, pour the orange sauce over the top and pass the french beans and giblet rice.

And if rain is forecast for Sunday, don't forget to set the clock.

Pheasant for a Peasant

Drop a bouillon cube in a cup of hot water and when it dissolves pour it into the bottom of a casserole. (That was the hard part.)

Cut the pheasant into serving-sized pieces, sprinkle with salt and pepper and place in the bouillon. Melt a cube of butter, stir in a quarter cup of flour until smooth, then let cool slightly until it begins to resemble library paste. Then spread it thickly over the pheasant pieces. When you've used it all up, sprinkle paprika over everything in sight and shove the casserole into a 350 oven. The bird should be done in an hour.

Giblet Rice

A side dish for any creature with surplus giblets. Toss the duck, chicken or turkey gizzard, neck and heart into a pan of salted water. Cook at a slow bubble for 90 minutes. Add the liver, cook another 10 to 15 minutes, and remove from heat. Drain and chop the gizzard, heart and liver into small pieces. Do the same to the meat you remove from the neck.

Saute 1/2 cup chopped onions and 1/4 cup chopped green pepper in two tablespoons butter until soft. Add 1/4 teaspoon salt, 1/8 teaspoon thyme and some freshly ground pepper.

At this point you can add either a cup of natural brown rice or a cup of quick brown rice to the pan, and stir until mixed with the onions and pepper.

If you use the natural rice, transfer to casserole, add three cups chicken bouillon, the giblets, cover and bake an hour in 350 oven.

If you use the quick rice you'll need add only two cups of chicken stock (and the giblet meat). Cover and cook for 30 minutes.

Meat Dishes

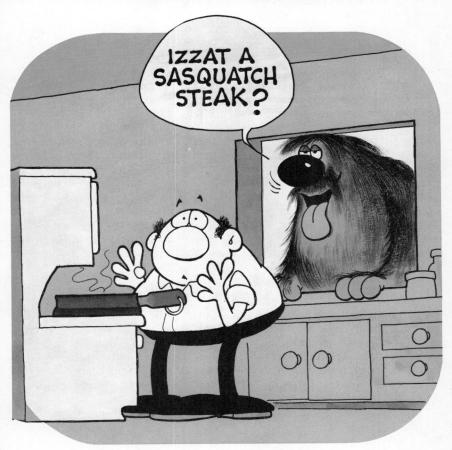

Certainly, I believe in the Sasquatch. Oh, yeah, I know that Sasquatch scare a couple of years ago in Eastern Washington was supposedly the work of a mischievious Colville bricklayer. But personally, I find it easier to believe in a half-man, half-beast than the spectacle of a Colville bricklayer running through the woods with lumber nailed to his shoes. Now that's weird!

Besides, I want to believe in the Sasquatch. I also believe in flying saucers, Alfred E. Newman and tenderloin of beef.

Of course, nobody has actually seen a tenderloin of beef since 1961, when the price rose to $37.50 a pound. But the memory lingers, and you'll occasionally encounter a recipe which begins:

"Have your butcher cut a loin steak three inches thick . . . "

The author then proposes you rub it with anchovy paste or roquefort cheese. This is a little like issuing a sweat shirt and dirty sneakers to the Playmate of the Month. (The Playmate of the Month is actually a Chewelah plumber in a remarkable disguise.)

If it actually exists, a tenderloin of beef needs no accessories, save possibly a touch of salt, pepper and flame, in inverse order.

However, ground chuck needs a little help, and there is nobody in America who will today dispute the existence of ground chuck. Bathed in a little red wine, it can even emerge as a suitable fare for guests.

But first a quick side dish:

Parmesan Rice

Peel and chop one onion and saute in 1/4 cup butter. When soft and golden, pour in one cup of white rice (No! No! Not minute rice!) Stir-cook until it begins to turn golden.

Pour in one cup chicken bouillon, one cup water, 1/4 cup sherry. Bring to a boil, cover, reduce heat to low and simmer 25 minutes.

Remove cover from pan, stir in 1/2 cup Parmesan cheese, two tablespoons butter, and serve with the:

Sasquatch Steak

Mince a clove of garlic and saute it lightly along with a scant cup of minced onion in two tablespoons butter. When the onion is transparent, plop it in a bowl and add:

1-1/2 lbs. ground chuck
1-1/2 tea. salt
Good pinch of thyme
2 T. soft butter
A grinding of fresh pepper
One egg.

Maul ingredients in bowl until thoroughly mixed, then form into cakes, coat with flour and saute in two tablespoons butter, in hot pan, until done. Keep the patties in a warm oven while you mess up some more pans.

Boil a mixture of 1/2 cup beef bouillon and 2/3 cup red wine in a small saucepan.

Pour the fat out of the frying pan and toss in two tablespoons minced green onion. Add the bouillon-wine mixture to the frying pan and boil rapidly, scraping the bottom of the pan with a wooden spoon.

When the mixture has boiled down to about a half cup, remove from the heat and stir in one teaspoon cornstarch blended with one teaspoon water. Return to heat and simmer one minute. Add salt and pepper, pour sauce over meat and serve immediately, maybe with some oven-heated onion rings, the rice and a salad which includes the anchovies and roquefort cheese you didn't rub on the tenderloin of beef.

And since you used less than a cup of the red wine on the Sasquatch Steak, chances are a thimbleful still remains in the jug.

BRZFLECK! (That's Sasquatch, for Skoal!)

I think it's my favorite part of the story, "A Christmas Carol." Ebenezer Scrooge throws open the window on that bright winter morning and shouts:

"Boy! You there, boy!"

"Me, sir?"

"Yes, you. What day is this?"

"Lor, Gov'nor, it's Christmas Day."

"Tell me, is that big package of ground beef still hanging in the butcher shop window?

"You mean the four-pound package of extra-lean ground beef? Yes sir, I saw it only this morning."

"Then fetch it for me. And there's a tuppence for you, if you deliver it to Bob Cratchit's house, at once."

Of course, that's the abridged version of the story. I think there used to be a goose or a turkey or a swan hanging in the butcher's window, in the original manuscript. Granted, Ebenezer Scrooge was L-O-A-D-E-D, but he'd have stayed home and shared a can of Spam with Christmas-Yet-To-Come before he'd pay today's prices for a bird. And as for a crab cocktail!

Lemme tell you about crab cocktail.

The Intermediate Eater's favorite cartoonist, Ray Collins, once gave me this super recipe for an economical crab cocktail, handed on to him by his sister. OK, crab cocktail for the special feast, right? It called for only one can and what could that cost, a buck and a quarter on the outside?

The first store I hit had only one brand — Formosa snow crab, for $1.80. Wait a minute. I'm living in the heart of Dungeness crab country and in the closest state to Alaska. I've got to send to Formosa for some snow crab? Not likely.

The next supermarket had some sort of Alaskan canned crab, but my elbow locked when I attempted to lift it off the shelf. The price read $3.25. No, no, not for a crab boat. Just for one crummy little can this big! I decided the third supermarket might be the charm.

Some charm! One (1) lousy (lousy) little can of Alaskan king crab was priced at $4.69. And you thought Tiny Tim knew how to cry!

So you're not getting the crab cocktail recipe, after all. And you're not getting a recipe for 10 bucks worth of stuffed swan, or whatever. We herewith present the Bah Humbug Holiday Feast.

Cheapo Cocktail

To serve six, buy a half pound of fresh mushrooms, wipe clean, slice.

Mix a half-cup catsup with a tablespoon of vinegar and 1/2 teaspoon prepared horseradish. Chill this topping until you are ready to serve. Slice the mushrooms atop some shredded lettuce in cocktail cups. Top with the sauce. Use it sparingly, if you like the taste of mushrooms. If you detest mushrooms, go heavy on the sauce.

Now the main course of the feast.

Christmas Logs

Again to serve six, you'll need about 2-1/2 pounds of lean ground beef. Form into 12 portions and flatten.

Mix some packaged dressing with the recommended moisture and half an onion, minced.

Put some dressing atop each patty and roll into logs.

Space out in oven dish and place in a 400 oven.

Mix over low heat two cans mushroom soup, four tablespoons of chili sauce, one tablespoon Worcestershire sauce and several drops of Tabasco.

After a half hour remove logs from oven and pour off grease. Slop the mushroom sauce over the logs and return to the oven for another 30 minutes.

Strawberry Mousse

In the event Christmas happens to fall in July use fresh strawberries (two cups) and mix with 3/4 cup of sugar. Otherwise, thaw some already-sweetened frozen berries. In either event, mix with 1/8 teaspoon salt and 1-1/2 teaspoons vanilla.

Whip one cup of cream and fold it into the berry mixture. Freeze until firm.

Let the freezer tray sit out at room temperature about 15 minutes before you plan to serve dessert.

And God bless us, every one. Even though crab is $4.69 a can.

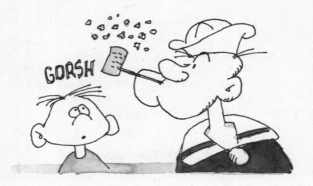

Personally, I think spinach has been given a bum rap and Popeye just may be to blame. A generation of parents raised their children to believe that if they ate their spinach, they'd be as strong as Popeye. I don't believe they ever took a good look at the gentlemen in question.

Granted, he had a pretty good left hook. He also had one eye, several tatoos, a questionable chin, a sailor suit, a build like a Polish sausage gone bad, and he occasionally consumed his spinach through the pipe he was forever sucking.

Obviously, a gentleman of discriminating taste.

He also occasionally opened the can with his teeth, endearing him to orthodontists far and wide.

I don't even want to bring up his girl friend Olive Oil. Suffice it to say that Brussels sprouts never had this image problem.

In any event, the hard sell had a predictable effect. The children decided that spinach tasted like Popeye's pipe or, worse yet, could possibly be good for you. Now adults, they nourish this inane aversion, announcing smugly that, "I don't like spinach," and admitting in the same breath that they haven't tasted it since Mussolini invaded Ethiopia.

Fresh spinach, served with a sprinkling of salt and a dollop of butter, is excellent fare even if it doesn't do much for your muscles. Some of the frozen varieties are almost as good. And even if you are not a real big canned spinach fan, it will serve adequately in an excellent meatball recipe which (in honor of u-know-who) could be called:

Sweet Pea's Meatballs

1 lb. ground chuck
1 cup cooked spinach
1 mashed clove garlic
1/2 cup grated parmesan
1 egg
1/2 tea. oregano
1 tea. salt
1/2 cup bread crumbs

Beat the egg with a fork and add to the ground chuck. Whether you use fresh, frozen or canned cooked spinach, drain it of excess fluid and add it to the bowl. Toss in the oregano, garlic, salt and parmesan, massage everything together for a minute or two, and then form into golf-ball sized meatballs. You should have about 15.

Roll the meatballs in the bread crumbs and place them in a lightly greased pan or large Pyrex baking dish. Bake in a 375 oven for about 25 minutes.

Although the meatballs are not cooked in a sauce, they emerge relatively moist, eminently eatable and should satisfactorily serve four.

If someone in the family maintains they dislike spinach, and asks, "Hey, what's this weird green stuff in the meatballs?" remark casually that it is no doubt a deadly fungus.

If they think it's bad for them, they'll probably eat it.

Meat Ball Stew

Mix a pound of hamburger with one slightly beaten egg, a half cup of bread crumbs, 1/4 cup of tomato sauce, a teaspoon of salt, 1/8 teaspoon pepper, 1/8 teaspoon allspice and 1/2 teaspoon onion powder.

Squish the mixture into about a dozen meatballs. Heat two tablespoons of oil in a heavy pot or deep frying pan and brown the meatballs on all sides.

Dump in three cups of water, 3/4 cup of tomato sauce, three peeled and cubed potatoes, about a cup and a half of sliced carrots, a green pepper cut in strips (after the white pith and seeds have been removed) and finally pour an envelope of dry onion soup mix over the top.

Bring the stew to a boil, stir a couple of times, reduce heat, cover the pot and let it simmer for about 30 minutes.

There are two ways to approach this supermarket shopping gig — the right way and the hungry way.

Say you put away a mouthful of coffee grounds for breakfast and gulped down a snow cone and a gingersnap for lunch, then along about 5:15 you grab a supermarket cart and begin the week's shopping. That's the wrong way, because you are hungry enough to eat the legs off the Jolly Green Giant display over there by the string beans.

And your battle plan proceeds like this:

"Hmmmm, these Spanish olives would go good with some of those watermelon pickles, and how about a can or two of anchovies, provided I can locate a few cartons of Snax-Crax."

By the time you get to the meat case your cart is loaded down with seven frozen pizzas, a German chocolate cake, two jars of quail eggs and $37.43 worth of Misc., and all you're going to be able to afford for dinner is two pounds of ground beef. Ergo, the family is going to find itself staring at some:

Beefo Cheapo

1/2 cup celery tops
1 chopped onion
2 lbs. ground beef
1 tea. salt
2 cans tomato soup
small can mushroom pieces
pinch cayenne
pinch thyme
pinch sage
pepper
3 T. parsley

Heat a tablespoon of butter at a medium setting in your skillet or electric frying pan. Toss in the chopped celery tops, the onion, cayenne and herbs and saute until soft.

Form the beef into an inch-thick slab, sprinkle both sides with salt and pepper. Plunk it into the pan, top with the mushroom bits and cook uncovered for 20 minutes.

Squash the meat down with a spatula, cook another 15 minutes, add the undiluted soup and parsley, stir, cook five minutes more, and serve with mashed potatoes or some noodles cooked in salted water.

Beefo Cheapo makes an entirely satisfactory meal. But if you had done the week's shopping after a bowl of minestrone and a large pepperoni pizza, your entire philosophy would have been transformed.

"Let's see, need something for dinner. (Urp.) Don't want any of those. Lord, can't think of eating one of them. Macaroni and spaghetti? (Belch). Oh, brother, I think I can skip this aisle altogether!"

By the time you arrive at the meat counter your basket contains a roll of Tums, a can of tuna and a half-pint of skim milk and you can afford two pounds of round steak to construct:

$wiss $teak

2 lbs. round steak
2 T. butter
1 can tomato sauce
1/2 tea. chili powder
1/4 cup lemon juice
1 tea. salt
1 tea. Worcestershire
flour
1 sliced onion
1/2 tea. dry mustard
1 cup tomato juice
1 tea. sugar
few shakes tabasco

Cut steak into serving-sized pieces, coat generously with flour. Brown in butter over medium high heat, turning once. While the meat is browning, fling all remaining ingredients in a bowl.

Reduce heat, pour contents of bowl over the steak, cover and simmer two hours or until tender.

If you put away a superburger at 11:30, but it's been three hours since lunch and you arrive at the supermarket starting line with a question mark in your stomach that's another story altogether.

Purchase a bottle of fine Portuguese Madeira from your wine merchant and you do not expect — upon the uncorking — to discover that you have actually been issued some Bubble-Up in disguise.

A guy anticipating a dry martini will develop a tic, if the first sip proves to be Guinness Stout.

No jury in the world would convict the assassin of a chef who persisted in adding chopped figs to the Oysters Rockefeller, or spreading liver paste on his angel food cakes.

But why can't this unwritten quality control be extended to other culinary corners, before we all fall to the ground clutching protesting stomachs?

Consider, for beginners, Exhibit A, otherwise known as Spanish Rice. OK, there it is, staring up at you from the cookbook or menu. Well, what is it?

It could be a lobster-and-prawn paella which would reduce a millionaire matador to sobs of appreciation. Or it could turn out to be a glutinous gut-buster constructed of two parts minit-rice and one part tomato catsup, with a handful of aged peas thrown in for color and character.

Consider Italian lasagne, because I'd rather not. You can anticipate only one certainty. It will contain several broad noodles, unless the chef happened to be out of broad noodles. It might emerge as an artful blend of beef, cheeses and spices. Another version, under the same name, could also be used to stucco the basement.

Chances are excellent that Beef Stroganoff will contain beef, although it might be sirloin cubes, ground chuck or an old ox joint. Another essential is sour cream, but these days a wandering chef might instead stir in yogurt, cottage (gasp) cheese or a shot glass of evaporated milk.

The injustices done to Hungarian Goulash were at least partially responsible for the 1848 revolution and the eventual fall of the Hapsburg Monarchy. I believe the first president of the Republic, Mihaly Karolyi, was elected on a platform specifying three tablespoons of paprika. He probably had something like this in mind:

Hungarian Goulash

3 T. shortening
2 buds garlic
3 lbs. lean beef cubes
3 T. paprika
2 cups beef bouillon
4 sprigs celery leaves
3 onions
1 tea. marjoram
1 tea. salt
2 T. tomato paste
4 sprigs parsley

Heat shortening in a saucepan and add the thinly sliced onions. Saute slowly until translucent. Add the chopped garlic, marjoram and cook five minutes more. Add the beef cubes, salt, paprika, stir the whole schmeer, cover and cook 30 minutes at a slow simmer.

Stir in tomato paste, bouillon, celery and parsley. Bring to a boil, then lower heat again to a simmer and cook, covered, for an hour. Remove and discard the celery tops and serve the meat and sauce atop hot, salted egg-noodles.

And before we leave the country you might consider:

✳ Hungarian Cabbage *Yummy*

A big head of cabbage will serve four. Chop it finely, discarding the core, and let it stand mixed with a tablespoon of salt for 30 minutes.

Rinse the cabbage in a collander under running water and then squeeze until relatively dry.

Melt a cube of butter in a large frying pan. Toss in the cabbage and cook uncovered over medium heat for 30 minutes, stirring frequently. Sprinkle the cabbage with three tablespoons sugar and some freshly ground pepper. Continue cooking, and occasionally stirring, about 15 minutes more, until cabbage begins to brown, and turn crip-sey. If it isn't crip-sey, it isn't genuine Hungarian Cabbage.

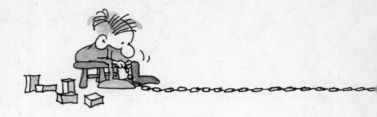

The wonders of modern education. Not too many years ago, it was possible to flunk geography by coloring Costa Rica green. Nicaragua was supposed to be green, Costa Rica orange. But if you were stuck with a dull crayon, Costa Rica's national boundaries were suddenly threatened, to say nothing of its self-determination.

Those were also the days when any artistic aspirations could be crushed instantly and finally by a part-time art teacher, who informed you that your soap sculpture of a graceful gazelle resembled a pregnant warthog. So you spent the remainder of the year constructing a 2.5-mile long chain out of paper clips, during the hour devoted to creative expression.

Today's students are not so instantly dismissed as artistic bummers. You mess up Costa Rica and the teacher has an explanation. It's simply that your "small muscles" have not yet developed. Of course the gazelle still looks like a warthog, but the teacher has issued a convenient copout.

The fact of the matter is that there are a lot of middle-aged men still standing around, waiting for their small muscles to develop. Give 'em a shovel or a lawn mower, and they create relatively little damage. But they can destroy a television set or a washing machine in 11.37 seconds with an 85-cent screwdriver.

And a lot of them shy away from can-openers and paring knives because somewhere along the way they encountered a Julia Child recipe that began:

"Skin and bone a small kangaroo with a double-edged razor blade . . ."

Cooking doesn't have to be all that complicated, but you've got to pick your shots. You can whip up a perfectly acceptable repast with the culinary equivalent of a shovel or rake. Then, ever so often, you can test the development of your small muscles with something just slightly more challenging, like maybe:

Beefeaters

Buy a two-pound hunk of sirloin or top round steak. If it's thick, you should slice it into two thin hunks of meat. Keep cutting until you have 12 pieces of meat of about equal size. Flatten them with a Hank Aaron-autographed Little League bat, and sprinkle with salt and pepper.

Combine 3/4 pound of high-grade sausage meat with three tablespoons chopped parsley and 1 minced garlic clove. Gloop some of the sausage mixture atop each slice of beef. Roll and tie each beefeater with a couple of pieces of string. This isn't as difficult as it sounds.

In a large frying pan heat two tablespoons butter and one tablespoon oil until mixture bubbles. Add the beef rolls and brown lightly on all sides. Stir in one cup sliced carrots and 1/2 cup sliced onions and cook several minutes.

Add 1/3 cup dry white wine and continue cooking four minutes. Add one and a half cups beef bouillon and two tablespoons tomato paste (or catsup). Cover pan and cook over low heat about 90 minutes.

Place meat on a warm platter. Skim fat from pan and serve the remaining sauce, unstrained, with the Beefeaters, whipped potatoes and a salad.

Hey . . . You . . . Stupid! You were supposed to remove the string from the rolls before you poured sauce all over them. Maybe you'd better stick to paper clips, and kitchen tasks less demanding, like:

Ranchhouse Roundsteak

Cut a top round steak into strips, sprinkle with salt and pepper, then toss lightly in flour. Brown in oil in hot pan, reduce heat and add two cans beef broth, one can water, one-quarter cup sherry, a can of mushroom pieces and one-third cup of grated romano cheese. Simmer about an hour and a half, until tender, and serve with rice or noodles. If you like a thicker sauce, mix some cornstarch with a bit of water and stir in just before serving.

Did it ever occur to you that parsnips actually do taste awful? Of course, children have been maintaining this for eons, but the scientific argument usually proceeds like this:

"Eat your parsnips, they're good."

"Are not!"

"Are too!"

"Are not!"

And the "are nots" usually prevail.

As adults, we have always assumed that our tastes are more cultivated, and consequently superior. Did it ever occur to you that a peanut butter and jelly sammich might be the gastronomical superior of pate de foie gras? And that martinis actually come off second best to lukewarm cocoa?

The thing that makes me wonder about this is an item I stumbled across some time ago while perusing either Gray's Anatomy, the writings of Herophilus of Chalcedon or possibly the inside of a matchbook. If I remember correctly, the item claimed that young children possess twice as many taste buds as mature adults. It seems that as we grow older, our taste buds are constantly being pickered off, one by one.

If this is true, are toddlers actually the gourmets of the world? Is cherry Kool-Aid intrinsically superior to a fine chablis? Does everything taste better soaked in chocolate syrup? Should licorice ice cream replace the after-dinner brandy and Havana cigar, in discriminating clubs.

I mean, how are parents going to win any arguments concerning spinach, calves liver and pigs knuckles if their offspring can counterattack with a superior epiglotis?

Maybe we'd better try to discourage future scientific speculation by concentrating on the few areas of agreement between the family provider, and the providees.

Teriyaki steak may be one such area, and the following is an excellent variation on same:

Tastebud Teriyaki

Select a medium-sized flank steak, to serve four. Plop it on your carving board and with a sharp butcher knife cut the steak in thin diagonal slices, across the grain. No! No! Don't cut it all the way through. You just want to butterfly it.

Next cut the flank steak into four serving pieces, and let them wallow around for about an hour in a mixture consisting of 1/4 cup soy sauce, a minced clove of garlic, one beaten egg and one-half teaspoon grated ginger root. (You can use dried ginger but gee, Gloria, it won't be the same.)

Mix one-half cup bread crumbs and one-half cup flour, coat the meat on both sides in this mixture and pan fry in hot oil until golden brown on both sides. This will take about eight to 10 minutes if you like your steak medium rare. And you should, if there's one healthy taste bud left in your epithelium.

You could serve the steak with a side dish of:

Deviled Carrots

6 large carrots
2 T. brown sugar
2 tea. dry mustard
1/2 cup butter
3 drops tabasco
1/2 tea. salt, pepper

Saute the carrots in the melted butter for about five minutes. Add the brown sugar, mustard, tabasco, salt and pepper. Cook 10 minutes and serve.

You say your kids don't like deviled carrots? Just explain to them logically:

"Shut up and eat your deviled carrots. They're good!"

Barbecue cooking in the Northwest contains certain intriguing elements of Russian roulette, particularly for the outdoor chef who cooks strictly by the book.

"Cook steak five minutes on each side over fairly hot charcoal fire," the recipe reads.

Only one thing wrong with those instructions. They were transcribed by a resident chef in Barstow, Calif., during an August afternoon when the hubcaps on his Volvo were melting in the driveway.

Follow these same culinary specifications on a chill afternoon in Bellevue, when a 15-mile-an-hour breeze is rustling the leaves and a sneeze seems imminent from that passing cloud, and the resultant beef-steak will resemble an Eskimo's moccasin after a walrus hunt.

Sure, some outdoor chefs may invest $50 in an imported hibachi with a lid like a bank vault door, in search of uniform cooking conditions. But the average backyard amateur is still cooking out of a rusting tripod which was obtained in exchange for one book of green stamps the year the family took Gramps to the rest home in Portland.

It is capable of barbecuing a nice batch of spare ribs in exactly 57 minutes, give or take two hours. The barbecued salmon will be ready in 35 minutes if the rain holds off, and 53 minutes if it doesn't. A chicken needs just 62 minutes of preparation, unless it happens to be burned after 41 minutes.

Lord knows how long it'll take you to broil that flank steak medium rare. It's been sitting in the refrigerator, marinating, for 11 1/2 hours. It's two inches thick on one end and a half-inch thick on the other. The temperature outside is exactly 68 degrees, providing you live on a runway at Sea-Tac Airport, where the radio thermometer is located. And a monsoon is scheduled to hit in 27 minutes.

Difficult assignment? Not at all.

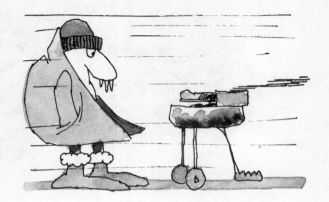

Frankly Flank Steak

With a sharp knife, score the flank steak lightly in five or six places on each side. Marinate overnight in 1/2 cup soy sauce, 2-1/2 tablespoons brown sugar, two tablespoons lemon juice, one teaspoon ground ginger and 1/2 teaspoon garlic salt.

Cook it outside a while OR retreat to kitchen, preheat the oven and broil three to four inches from the heat for about five minutes on each side. Cut in thin diagonal slices, serve on hot plates, and convert the barbecue cart into a planter.

You might want to prepare in advance a side dish of:

Rice and Peas

Melt 1/4 cup butter and a tablespoon olive oil in a heavy saucepan. Add one-half strip bacon, diced, and a chopped onion. Stir-cook until onion is soft and translucent.

Add a package of frozen peas, which have been allowed to partially thaw. Cook-stir five minutes. Add 3/4 cup raw rice and stir-cook three minutes. Add 1-3/4 cups chicken bouillon, 1/ teaspoon salt and some freshly ground pepper.

Cook covered over low heat for 15 to 20 minutes. Ladle the rice into a heated serving bowl, stir in a spoonful of grated parmesan cheese and serve with the steak slices and maybe some garlic bread in a kitchen or dining room thermostatically heated to 68 degrees. And close the window!

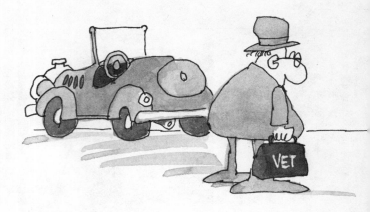

In his entertaining Cow Country Cook Book, a one-time cowpuncher named Dan Cushman recounts the tale of the Montana ranch hand who wandered into the Chequamegon Cafe in Butte and ordered a T-bone steak.

It arrived on a platter thick, hot and blood rare.

"Would you like me to bring the Bordelaise sauce?" the waitress asked after the cowpoke had taken the first hesitant slice with his knife.

"Gosh no," he responded. "Bring the linament. I think we may be able to save this one."

A well-done steak, on the other hand, is beyond repair, fit only to resole aged logger boots or to line a catcher's mitt. The Cult of the Beefeater dictates that a steak be served up blood-red on the inside, unadorned except for a whack of melting butter, salt and pepper. If you're inclined to order it otherwise, save your money and invest in a tunafish sandwich, cooked medium-well.

It is therefore sacrilegious to suggest that top sirloin be served up with a sauce, marinade or (croak) a pool of catsup. Since the average American wage-earner is able to invest in a choice cut of steak about as often as he dates Olga Korbut, why should he want it to taste like anything else? Anybody who eats steak so often it becomes a bore has to be cheating on his income tax and will shortly be investigated (and perhaps recalled) by Ralph Nader.

With that premise established, I'd like to suggest a super marinade for a choice steak. Since I already have my tax refund, I am obviously clean.

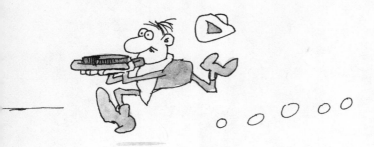

Steak Pepp-rika

Coarsely crush a tablespoon of peppercorns with a mortar and pestle (or some waxed paper and a ball-peen hammer). Toss the cracked pepper into a bowl and add two teaspoons of salt, two teaspoons of paprika, two teaspoons of crushed rosemary and two smashed cloves of garlic. Add one-quarter cup of olive oil and mix thoroughly.

This will be sufficient marinade for four to six choice steaks. Pour it over the meat and let it work its wonders for several hours, turning the meat once. Then broil the steaks only until they have passed the stage where linament is still a beneficial possibility.

You might serve the company steaks with:

Garlic Crouton Salad

Peel and halve two cloves of garlic and rub both sides of two thick slices of dry bread. Cut crusts off bread, dice into squares, let brown slightly in oven, then remove.

Wash and dry sufficient leaf lettuce. Break into pieces and chill, covered, in refrigerator. Immerse a fresh egg in boiling water for exactly one minute, then remove.

When ready to serve, place lettuce in a large salad bowl. Add 1/4 teaspoon dry mustard and 1/2 teaspoon each salt and pepper and toss. Add 1/2 cup olive oil and toss. Add two tablespoons wine vinegar and one teaspoon lemon juice and toss. Crack that half-cooked egg into the salad and toss again. Add croutons, toss a final time and serve . . . medium rare.

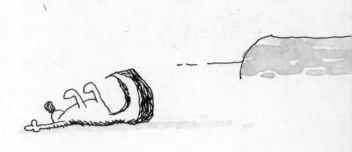

Research has established that it is possible to satisfactorily grill and serve an old logger boot, provided it has been marinated a suitable time in red wine. Unfortunately, I have misplaced the recipe for Grilled Logger Boot. I believe it specifies immersion in Chianti for approximately 19 months. At room temperature. (The laces are cooked al dente, in boiling water, and tossed lightly with parmesan cheese.)

A chuck roast requires slightly less preparation, and also tastes better. In fact, if your barbecue guests aren't too bright, you might be able to convince them they're getting steak. The trick is to marinate the roast, grill it medium rare over hot coals, and then carve into thin slices with a sharp knife.

Or you can eliminate these three steps and your guests will swear they are being served authentic Filet Thom McAn. Well done.

There are countless excellent marinades, but make sure that yours includes one of the tenderizing agents like vinegar, lemon juice or wine. Purchase a round bone roast, let it vegetate for at least 24 hours in the marinade, and you are ready to heat up the barbecue.

Logger Boot Marinade

Mix together one cup red wine, 1/2 cup salad oil, one-third cup brown sugar, 1/4 teaspoon salt, 1/4 teaspoon marjoram, 1/4 teaspoon rosemary, one mashed clove of garlic and a few drops of tabasco. Slice two onions; add to the marinade and then pour the whole schmeer over the roast and refrigerate. Turn it a few times during the 24-hour bath and remove from refrigerator about an hour before you intend to barbecue it. A two-inch-thick roast, cooked about 12 minutes on each side over a hot fire, will slice rare. You may want to grill it a bit longer but don't overcook.

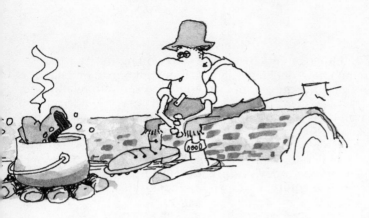

Another Merciful Marinade

Mince two cloves garlic and saute gently in two tablespoons oil. (Olive oil is best, peanut oil is satisfactory, but you'll probably use vegetable oil.) Add 1/4 teaspoon dry mustard, 1/2 teaspoon crushed rosemary and one teaspoon soy sauce. Remove from heat and stir in two tablespoons wine vinegar and four tablespoons dry white wine.

Pour sauce over roast in bowl and refrigerate 24 hours, turning occasionally. An hour before dinner time, remove the meat from the bowl, and add to the marinade two tablespoons catsup, 1/2 teaspoon Worcestershire sauce and two teaspoons steak sauce. Stir well and spread this on the roast before you toss it on the grill. Turn meat frequently and baste often.

You could serve it with a tossed green salad. (Try sprinkling the salad generously with shelled sunflower seeds.) And pass the French bread.

Franco-Italian Bread

Cut a loaf of French bread into one-inch slices, but don't cut all the way through the bottom crust. Mince two cloves garlic, add to one cube softened margarine, 1/4 teaspoon paprika and 1/4 cup parmesan cheese. Smear this mixture on each slice of bread, wrap the loaf in aluminum foil and heat (until piping hot) on back of the barbecue grill or in the oven. If you heat it on the grill, turn it occasionally or the crust will burn and taste like the sole of an old logger boot.

There really shouldn't be much surprise surrounding the fact that so many American men have decided to grab a butcher knife in one hand, a pod of garlic in the other and mount an attack on the refrigerator and stove.

These days a guy has to have some excuse for hanging around the house, and cooking is one of the few legitimate ones left.

By tradition, the male of the family is also the resident handy-man and all-round Mister Fixit. Hollow laughter. What's to fix?

If the machines running today's household decide to revolt (and they will, every 23 months by mutual accord) immediate surrender is recommended.

Take the back off your color television set and you violate your warranty, your life insurance and are also required to mail a $25 check to the estate of David Sarnoff. A furnace which begins to send up Apache smoke signals between muffled explosions is not the proper subject for a study of Beginning Electronics.

Armed with nothing more than a screwdriver, you can wreck $62.37 worth of damage in just 11 minutes on a clothes dryer that needs a 23-cent whatzit.

And once the dishwasher notices this obvious truth, it begins spitting out cocktail forks on alternate revolutions.

What can you do with a 30-gallon water tank when it developes a 40-gallon leak? Give it a transfusion?

Oh, sure, the opportunity will occasionally arise to change a lightbulb or to deliver a healing kick to a singing toilet. But these tasks award possibly less artistic or creative satisfaction then Michelangelo's Apollo or the invention of the cavity magnetron oscillator.

But take cooking, as an alternative.

OK, you start with maybe $1.90 worth of sirloin or sukiyaki beef. Toss in a few onions, a green pepper, a few sips of this and a slop of that. Following simple instructions you are probably going to be able to whip up some acceptable Sherry-Soy Steak. But what if you do weld it to the frying pan or pour it down the side of the stove by mistake? You can't buy the button that turns on the refrigerator light for $2.77.

Following are the manufacturer's specifications. Replacement parts do not have to be mail-ordered from Ann Arbor, Mich.

Sherry-Soy Steak

1 1/2 lbs. sirloin or sukiyaki beef, cut 1/4 inch thick. You'll also need:

5 T. vegetable oil
2 T. Sherry
2 T. soy sauce
2 T. cornstarch
1 green pepper
1/2 tea. sugar
3 onions
1 bud garlic

Peel and slice the onions. Slice pepper in strips, discarding white pith. Heat half the oil in frying pan or Chinese wok and saute the onions, green pepper and a minced clove of garlic three minutes. Add the sugar, one tablespoon soy sauce and one tablespoon sherry. Stircook briefly, then remove onion-pepper mixture to a warm plate.

Toss the meat with cornstarch and remaining soy sauce and sherry. Heat remaining oil in pan and brown steak. Return onion-pepper mixture to pan, stir-fry another two minutes and serve, maybe with some brown rice.

Steak and Pods

Buy a pound of snow pea pods when they're in season. You'll also need 1 1/2 pounds of sirloin steak or sukiyaki beef. If you spot a special on mushrooms, grab a cup, since it hardly costs more to go first class. Assembly also:

3 T. sherry
3/4 cup veg. oil
2 garlic buds
2 T. cornstarch
1/2 cup soy sauce
1 tea. sugar

Cut the meat into thin strips, if you didn't buy it already prepared. Toss with the sherry, two tablespoons soy sauce and the cornstarch. Let this stand about 20 minutes.

You might have to remove the strings from the snow peas, but if they are young and tender this is unnecessary. Cook the pea pods about three minutes in boiling water, then drain.

Heat 1/2 cup oil in skillet. Saute beef until brown, along with the washed and sliced mushrooms, in the event you were a big spender. Heat remaining oil in second skillet and saute snow peas two minutes. Toss the beef into this pan, along with the minced garlic, the sugar and remaining soy sauce, mix well and serve when hot, maybe with boiled rice.

What's that? You say your stove burner is smoking and tossing sparks at the cat? I got my own problems, Clyde!

111

Mind, you, I really liked that drama at the Seattle Playhouse. The cast was superior, the plot provoking, the dialogue clever and unpredictable.

But I was slightly distracted by the chicken. It wasn't the fault of the playwright, or the cast. It's just one of my foibles.

See, they brought in this bucket of Col. Sanders' chicken in the first act and disappeared off stage with it, announcing that they're going to keep it warm in the oven.

Well, they forgot about it until the third act. They forgot. I didn't. While the actors were threatening to shoot each other, or worse, I kept thinking about that chicken in the oven, drying up, or worse.

Say I'm watching a drama on television, or at a movie. The husband and wife are sipping champagne in this fancy restaurant. The waiter sweeps up to the table, bearing an expensive silver tray, and places two orders of snails, in garlic butter, in front of these gracious diners.

The wife digs one nummy out with her cocktail fork, chews on it meditatively, then says:

"Lawrence, I think you should know I've been sleeping with Count Morcy."

"You've been what?"

"I know it's a shock." Sob.

The sob is mine. 'Cause there go the snails, in garlic butter.

If she is bound she's going to proclaim a marital crisis, why in chutney can't she do it after they've disposed of the snails? How can anybody worry about Count Morcy when the snails are getting cold? If she had waited through the snails, shared a Chateaubriand and a bottle of bourdeaux, the female in the drama would most likely have sighed, belched softly, and told herself:

"Oh, well, what he doesn't know won't hurt him. What's for dessert?

And it would sure help my piece of mind.

During gunfights, infidelity and the conquest of nations, I worry that they're broiling the steak too long, letting the ice cream melt or the gravy congeal.

The latter qualifies as a positive dramatic disaster, particularly if there is lots of gravy, served up hot with pot roast and mashed potatoes.

Mexican Pot Roast

Actually, it's supposed to be a Swedish pot roast. But I was out of cognac. Matter of fact, I've been out of cognac for about five years. So I substituted some light Mexican rum. You'll need:

3 to 4 lb. pot roast
4 T. butter
1 chopped onion
2 cups hot water
4 T. molasses
1/4 tea. allspice
1 T. vinegar
1-1/2 cups half and half
2 tea. salt
pepper
2 sliced carrots
1/4 cup rum
1/4 tea. basil
2 tea. anchovy paste
2 T. flour

Rub the roast with salt and pepper. Toss the butter into whatever cooking pot you're using and when it is sizzling, brown the meat on all sides. Add the onions and carrots and cook 10 minutes under medium heat, stirring occasionally.

Dump in two cups of hot water, the rum, molasses, basil, allspice, anchovy paste and vinegar.

Cook, covered, over low heat or in 300 oven for 2-1/2 hours. Plunk meat onto a warm platter, and let it coast. Mix the half and half with the flour and stir it into the gravy in a slow stream. Cook five minutes, just below boiling point, stirring as it thickens.

Serve hot, moist slices of the pot roast, small mountains of mashed potatoes, with gravy splashed liberally over everything.

And if your wife starts to interrupt your nice dinner, give her six bits and tell her to go eat a Big Mac with Count Morcy.

Under cross examination, I must admit I am not a pillar of strength during a meat boycott. Oh, I might have a couple of scrambled eggs with kippers for breakfast and a tuna sammich for lunch, but I usually head straight for purgatory along about 6:15.

I might be willing to boycott beef, except that I can't afford crab, shrimp, scallops or salmon, and if you think I'm going to make do with an ersatz lamb chop manufactured out of pulverized soybeans and used inner tubes you are entitled to one more guess.

However, I do know how the price of beef can be reduced across the board, without controls or fines, and eliminating the necessity of mailing a pound of ground chuck to Henry Jackson.

All this country has to do is to hire The Banana Man, and put him in charge of sirloin steak.

I don't actually know his identify. But he is . . . well, he's The Man in charge of Bananas.

My wife swears on a stack of old newspapers that the price of bananas has been 12 cents a pound for the past 15 years (which immediately pegs her age at 16 or above.) And sometimes they are on special for a dime. (Bananas, not wives.)

Why is that? Granted, the pickers might learn a thing or two from Cesar Chavez, but aren't there some middlemen between the banana tree and me? How about the wage scale of longshoremen, maritime workers, teamsters? Doesn't it cost more to fuel a freighter between . . . err, Bananaland, and Seattle?

The Banana Man obviously has some kind of super swindle going and he should be encouraged to share the secret with a cowboy so we can all afford:

A Pot of Roast

Tear off a big hunk of aluminum foil. Put across the bottom of a large, flat oven dish. Plunk about a four-pound pot roast on top. Put it under the broiler and brown on all sides.

Meanwhile, finely chop four stalks of celery, do the same to five carrots and mince two peeled cloves of garlic. Dump all this on top of the roast, add salt and pepper. Fold the foil up around the sides of the meat. Pour in one cup of red wine, seal the foil and cook for two hours at 325. Open a small hole in the foil, pour in a half cup more of red wine, seal and cook for another 30 minutes. (Already, you know this recipe came from the California Wine Institute, right?)

Carefully fold the foil back from the top of the roast. Remove meat to a warm platter. Pour the wine and juices and all the vegetables into a saucepan. Mix some of this liquid with two tablespoons of flour in small bowl until smooth, then stir back into the saucepan over medium heat.

Serve the sliced pot roast with mashed potatoes and spoon the wine-vegetable gravy over everything, except the apple pie, which is for dessert.

If you ran amuck and used up all the gravy and don't have anything to go with the leftover roast tomorrow, try this recipe.

Second-Hand Cow

Melt two tablespoons of bacon fat or lard in a skillet. Add one chopped onion and one chopped clove of garlic and cook over low heat until onion turns golden.

Add the slices of meat to the skillet, along with a mixture composed of one teaspoon salt, one/quarter teaspoon pepper, two tablespoons Worcestershire Sauce, one tablespoon vinegar and four tablespoons chili sauce.

Cover the skillet and simmer everything for 15 minutes, adding a small amount of water if necessary. Serve with buttered noodles, a tossed salad and 12 cents worth of bananas.

The first trip to Europe worked out remarkably well, considering that it began with a prune wrapped in bacon. Since it was consumed at 30,000 feet after one martini, it seemed wise to solicit a second opinion. Fortunately, Tacoma sports editor Earl Luebker happened to be munching doubtfully on something two seats forward.

"Earl," I asked, "what do you suspect that was you just swallowed?"

"I'm afraid I just ate a prune wrapped in bacon," he responded, gulping twice.

The confirmation led to some silent speculation. Was this a new airlines ploy to discourage hijacking? It should at least discourage hijackers from eating unidentified hors d'oeuvres. There was another possible explanation. Was this a preview of the native food? The jet was headed for London. Was it possible that the English began every meal with a prune wrapped in bacon?

The answer was no. The English begin their meals with "starters" like egg mayonnaise, which proved to be half a hard-boiled egg residing in a puddle of calories. Then they eat peas and chips. Granted, the restaurants sometimes add a lamb chop, a slice of beef or some deep-fried plaice. But sure as there's a pigeon in Trafalger Square, deep fried potatoes and peas will occupy the other half of the plate.

Oh, that's not all the English eat. Between meals they snack on jellied eel and drink warm pop, which is really quite impressive. An inquisitive foreigner with a stomach of forged steel will back down in six seconds, after an eye-to-eye confrontation with a cupful of jellied eel.

Obviously, Englishmen would be long extinct if forced to subsist on their own cuisine. They don't. The busiest restaurants in London are those pumping out ersatz American food. The restaurants are called Old Kentucky, Texas Pancake House, Wimpy, Chuckwagon and Tennessee. The hamburgers only faintly resemble hamburgers except at a restaurant called The Great American Disaster, where the genuine article is purveyed. By Americans.

But the British really owe their robust appetites to Spanish immigrants, who seem to control the kitchens of London. Waiters in the French restaurants speak Spanish. The cooks in the Chinese restaurants speak Spanish. The waiters and cooks in the traditional English restaurants speak Spanish.

"You wan bacon-eg?" they inquire brightly each morning, at bed-and-breakfast hotels from Canterbury to York.

Oh, we did encounter one genuine British waiter in Chester. He hated Americans. Oh, not all Americans, he confided. "Just ones like that penny-farthing pig at the other table."

If you are not a farthing pig, you might enjoy a great meal at a restaurant featuring a British waiter and a Spanish chef who owns a French cookbook. He might serve up something like:

Henry VIII's Pot . . . Roast

Heat four tablespoons of cooking oil to smoking in a roasting pan and brown the pot roast on all sides. (This particular roast weighed 3-1/2 pounds.)

Pour off oil and transfer meat to oven casserole. Add one cup dry red wine, two cups beef bouillon, two minced cloves garlic and three-fourths of a cup each of chopped onions, sliced carrots and celery tops. Add two tablespoons chopped parsley, 1-1/2 teaspoons thyme and sprinkle generously with salt and pepper. Cover casserole and cook in a 325 oven for 3-1/2 hours.

Remove meat to a warm dish. Strain the liquids, return to the pan you originally used to brown the meat and set it atop a stove burner. Bring to a slow boil. Stir in one tablespoon cornstarch which has previously been mixed with water. Cook, stirring, until liquid thickens, then serve with the sliced pot roast. The flavor is great.

Might even kill the taste of that incredible prune, wrapped in bacon.

I have this theory which I really hate to publicize in this era of rising food prices. But I honestly think a guy can survive nicely, on three cents a day.

The three cents must be invested in a lapel badge, with stickum on one side and red lettering on the other reading:

HI, MY NAME IS . . .

Write "Clyde" in the open space, and you are in business. For the next nine months you can survive nicely on free booze, chicken livers wrapped in bacon, cashew nuts and anchovy-paste canapes, provided you confine your activities to hotel mezzanines.

Your, "Hi, My Name is Clyde" pin should admit you to cocktail parties sponsored by every convening organization from International Tinfoil to the USS Midway Cooks and Bakers Alumni Organization.

Actually, this isn't really a theory at all, but a proven fact. It was proven a couple of years ago when a sudden change in schedule allowed my wife and me to attend a Montana University alumni banquet at a local hotel.

We arrived at the proper room on the mezzanine, and were greeted by a guy fondling a highball glass.

"Are these the Grizzlies?" I asked.

"Rrrrouuuuggghhhh!" he responded. I knew we were in the right place.

Except that the drinks were on the house, which seemed somewhat unusual since the freight for the banquet was only about $5. My wife spotted a woman from Anaconda, but couldn't remember her name. I caught the glance of a Sigma Nu, but didn't know him very well.

But, what the hay! The drinks were free and when we arrived at the banquet table we were confronted by enormous crab cocktails and by a gentleman across the table who asked, "You with our Seattle office?"

We were not, it transpired, at a university alumni gathering, but rather at a convention of insurance adjusters. The Montana banquet had been shifted a few days earlier to another hotel, the drinks were $1.25 a pop and the first course was fruit cocktail.

There is only one trouble with living on mezzanines. After nine months you begin to look like somebody who has been putting away a lot of bourbon, chicken livers and anchovy paste and you should rush home for something more substantial like:

Grizzly-Bear Stew

2 onions
2 lbs. stew meat
1/4 lb. mushrooms
2 cups carrot chunks
1/2 cup red wine
2 potatoes
1/2 cup water
1/4 tea. basil
1 can tomato soup
salt, pepper, parsley

Peel and chop the onions and potatoes, then fling everything into a casserole or pot, cover, and shove into a 275 oven for five hours.

Hot Pot

2 lbs round steak
2 tea. Worcestershire
1 tea. parsley
1 T. vinegar
1/4 tea. pepper
3 quartered potatoes
1/2 tea. salt
4 diced turnips
1 diced onion
6 shakes tabasco
4 diced carrots

Cube the round steak and coat in seasoned flour. Shake off excess and brown meat in hot oil in skillet. Remove meat from pan, add a little water to the pan juices, stir a couple of times and let it simmer for a few minutes.

Pour this gravy into a pot or casserole. Add Worcestershire, parsley, salt, vinegar, tabasco and pepper. Fling the meat and the vegetables into the pot and add enough water to cover.

Cover and cook in a 300 oven for three hours, remove from oven and thicken with gravy with a flour-water mixture if you wish.

No, you don't have time for dessert. Some big spenders have ordered marinated shrimp and crab canapes sent up to the Rex Room at 6:15 and they'll go fast.

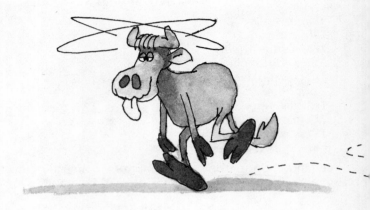

Reports have reached us that they do, indeed, have massage parlors in Japan. But I'm afraid the full story is less sensational than you might have hoped.

What they massage is cows. Beef cattle, to be exact.

Maybe it loses something in the translation, but we understand that what they do is back a steer into a stall, then a lot of nice ladies stand around and massage him (her? it?).

Can you imagine? "Oh, golly, just a little higher up on the flank steak," he sighs. "A little higher . . . there, there, that's it! Now scratch a little and then you can concentrate on the rump roast!"

It's not a religious rite at all. They are merely tenderizing the steer, on the hoof. Marinating the meat in vinegar might have the same eventual result, but obviously isn't nearly as much fun.

According to eyewitnesses, you can carve Kobe beef with a bread stick, but it also costs about three million yen (serves four).

Your average Seattle supermarket may currently be out of Kobe beef, although who knows? They have been peddling buffalo roasts and turkey burgers, so anything's possible. But if you do encounter some you'll probably find yourself short of yen.

As an alternative for supper, you can always massage some stewing beef, but don't let your neighbors catch you at it.

Actually, what you are doing is rubbing essential seasonings into the meat but it may also have a tenderizing effect, particularly if you subsequently cook hell out of it.

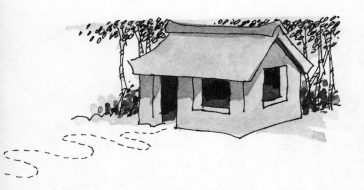

Massage Parlor Stew

For this particular stew, you begin by tossing one teaspoon of thyme into a mortar with one teaspoon of salt and 1/4 teaspoon of pepper. Grind the mixture thoroughly, then rub into the meat. Two pounds of stew meat will feed between four and six.

After rubbing with the seasoning, roll the meat lightly in flour, then set aside.

In a large pan saute a chopped onion in two tablespoons of butter plus one and a half tablespoons of cooking oil. When the onion becomes translucent and soft (not brown) remove from pan.

Turn up heat, brown meat well in the pan and then sprinkle it with 1-1/2 tablespoons of paprika. Return onion to pan, mix well and then remove from heat.

Add beef bouillon or broth until it just covers the meat and mix in two tablespoons of tomato paste. (Ya wanna use catsup? Use catsup!)

Simmer covered in your electric frying pan or in a 300 oven for an hour. Add four or five potatoes, peeled and diced, six carrots, peeled and sliced, then cover and cook for another 40 minutes.

Thicken sauce by mixing two tablespoons cornstarch with a little water, then stirring into the stew. Sprinkle with parsley, and serve.

Twenty minutes later one of your satisfied customers might even be willing to scratch your back.

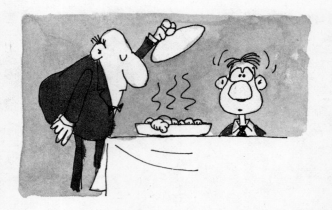

Betty Crocker calls them "variety meats" but the cowhands called them innards. And they concocted a tasty campfire dish containing liver, kidneys, hearts and sweetbreads which was commonly called S.O.B. Stew.

The term is seldom heard today. And most fine restaurants have invented a new culinary language to soft-peddle the news that they are serving up innards with their candlelight and soft wine.

Why? Nothing wrong with innards at all. Sweetbreads sauted with mushrooms are fantastic. Stuffed heart is the poor man's rib roast. Liver can be prepared deliciously a dozen different ways.

But some people have a tough time getting past the anatomical description. And I'll have to admit I go slow on brains and tongue.

For one thing, I find it personally impossible to attack a brain with a butcher knife. A paring knife looks too much like a scalpel and I'd momentarily expect a scream and a feminine voice at my shoulder shouting, "Doctor, not the cerebral cortex!"

An aversion to tongue can probably be traced to a youth misspent watching cows munch.

There I go, discouraging you from some new areas of culinary excitement. Actually, the intent was to encourage you to jazz up your next beef stew with a veal kidney, just for openers. Chances are nobody at the table will realize what they're eating. All they'll know is that it's good.

It is.

Really!

Son-a-Gun Stew

Trim the fat from a pound of beef stew meat and cut into bite-sized hunks. Do the same with the veal kidney, after trimming the white gristle. (Quit grinding your teeth, and trim the white gristle).

Coat the stew meat in flour and brown in butter or peanut oil. Chop one onion and fling it into the pan. Coat the hunks of kidney in flour, toss into the pan and stir-and-sizzle everything until the onion is getting limp and the meat is nicely browned.

Pour in one cup red wine, salt, pepper, one beef bouillon cube and a half teaspoon of rosemary. Add enough water to barely cover. Put a lid on the pan and simmer for two hours.

Add three sliced carrots and a handful of chopped parsley. Cover and cook another 30 minutes. Uncover and cook another 30 minutes, to thicken the gravy. (Total cooking time is thus three hours.)

Plop it on some mashed potatoes . . . What's that? You say you don't want kidneys in your stew. Scheeee! OK, then try this.

Bonneville Beef Stew

1/4 cup flour
1/4 tea. pepper
1/8 tea. ground cloves
1/4 cup margarine
1/2 cup red wine
1 can beef consomme
1/2 tea. salt
1/4 tea. thyme
2 lbs. stew meat
3 sliced onions
1 T. catsup

Mix the flour with the salt, pepper and spices. Coat the beef hunks evenly and reserve remaining flour.

Melt margarine in heavy skillet or electric frying pan, and saute meat until brown on all sides. Dump in the sliced onions and stir-cook until translucent.

Sprinkle the remaining flour and spices over the meat and onions. Add the consomme, wine and catsup, mooshing everything around with a wooden spoon.

Cover, reduce heat, and cook at a slow simmer for about 90 minutes.

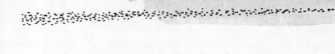

I want to tell you that T-H-E-Y knew how to throw a picnic!

Who, you well may ask, is T-H-E-Y?

The people who hung around with Mrs. John Sherwood, back in 1891. Their identities are lost in history, the memories faded by time. But you've gotta believe they went out in style, belching softly.

Recent research through microfilmed back copies of the newspaper was interrupted by a headline proclaiming, "Mrs. John Sherwood Tells How to Conduct a Picnic."

"The real picnic which calls for talent and executive ability should emanate from some country house where two or three other country houses shall cooperate and help. Then what jolly drives in the brake, what queer old family horses and antedeluvian wagons, what noble dog carts and what prim pony phaetons can join in the procession.

"The night before the picnic, which presumably starts early, the lady of the house should see to it that a boiled ham of perfect flavor is in readiness and she may flank it with a boiled tongue, four roasted chickens, a game pie and any amount of stale bread to cut into sandwiches.

"Claret is the favorite wine of picnicking, as being light and refreshing. Ginger ale is excellent and cheap. Champagne goes well with chicken and the more elaborate pate de foie gras. Some men prefer sherry with their lunch, some take beer. If you have room and a plentiful cellar, take all these things . . . "

That's what I always say, bring all these things!

But our society has progressed, since 1891. The Seattle housewife no longer spends Friday preparing for the feast. She isn't even home Friday, since she is chairman of a sub-committee of the League of Women Vultures, and Saturday morning at picnic time she'll hurl a brown paper bag in your direction. It contains a peanut-butter-and-jelly sammich, an aged carrot stick and a Twinkie.

Better you should let wild dogs roam Seward Park, while you stay home in the backyard and treat your family to some ribs.

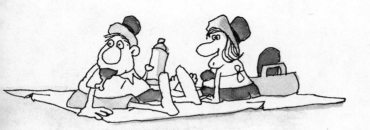

Backyard Spareribs

Let the spareribs simmer in salted water to cover for 30 to 45 minutes in advance, remove and pat dry.

Cut in serving-sized pieces and when barbecue fire is hot, toss the man-sized hunks on the grill, turning and basting frequently with a sauce made by combining one stick butter with 3/4 cup ketchup, 3 tablespoons lemon juice, 1/2 cup brown sugar, two teaspoons bottled steak sauce, two teaspoons hot pepper sauce, two teaspoons Worcestershire sauce and one tablespoon dijon-style mustard.

Cook until the ribs are crisp, but not charred. How long? That depends upon whether the temperature is 90 and the wind 10 miles per hour, or the temperature 10, and the wind 90.

Actually, if things turn that bad, you can stay inside, heating the oven to 350, sprinkling the unboiled ribs with salt, placing on rack in roasting pan, spreading with sauce and baking for a total of 90 minutes, basting after 30 minutes, then every 15 minutes until done. Serve the leftover basting sauce warm, in a gravy bowl, so people can pour it all over their ribs and create a great mess. The ribs go well with:

Caraway Potato Salad

Stir together a cup of mayonnaise; 1/4 cup sour cream, 1/4 cup milk, one minced clove garlic, 1 tablespoon caraway seed, 1-1/4 teaspoon salt and 1/8 teaspoon white pepper.

Boil and peel about six potatoes. Cut into cubes, mix with dressing while still warm, add more salt and pepper if needed and chill until the ribs are cooked. And pass the claret, champagne, sherry, beer . . . . . .

Tell the truth. How many kids do you know who want to grow up to be pig farmers?

I know the answer. Not a lot. Why is that? Why don't you ever see pig ranch foremen portrayed as motion picture heroes? Why is it that Zane Grey wrote about the cattle barons and the rival sheepmen and skipped the pig people altogether?

Did you ever plead with your father to let you take a summer vacation on a pig farm in Missouri? How many times have you seen John Wayne slopping the hogs? Did Charlie Russell ever complete a portrait of a pig? Does Johnny Cash sing ballads to Berkshires? Infrequently, you'll admit.

For every person in America there is somewhere half a hog running around a feed lot or sty, but you probably don't even care which end is yours. We worship the steer, must take a second mortgage on the power mower to finance a cubed steak, and only rarely make a supermarket charge for:

Pork Chops

1-1/2 lbs. chops
1 cup fine bread crumbs
1 T. chopped parsley
1 T. butter
salt, pepper
minced clove garlic
1 beaten egg
2 tea. water
3 T. olive oil
3/4 cup wine vinegar
flour

Trim excess fat from chops and marinate in the vinegar for an hour. Drain and pat dry.

Season the chops with salt, pepper. Dip each one in flour, coating both sides. Dip in the egg, which has been combined with two teaspoons of water. Finally, coat both sides in the bread crumbs, which have been mixed with the parsley and garlic.

Heat the olive oil and tablespoon butter in a skillet and brown the chops over medium heat for about five minutes on each side. If you're using an electric frying pan, lower heat to 280, cover and cook another 20 minutes. If you brown the chops in a regular skillet, cover and place in 300 oven for 20 minutes.

126

Chinese Pork Chops

6 chops
1 T. sugar
2 minced cloves garlic
2 T. applesauce
1-1/2 tea. salt
1/4 cup soy sauce
2 T. sherry
2 T. honey

Combine the sugar and salt. Take 3/4 tea. of mixture and rub on both sides of chops. Refrigerate two hours.

Brown chops over medium heat, approximately 10 minutes on each side. Pour off the fat.

Combine the garlic, soy sauce, sherry, applesauce, honey and remaining sugar-salt. Pour over the meat, cover and simmer over low heat for 40 minutes, basting occasionally.

Either dish should go great with some:

Pig Farm Potatoes

Cook six medium potatoes, until just done as tested with a fork. Skin, dice and add:

1/4 lb. diced cheese (Swiss or Monterey jack).
1 chopped onion
1/2 slice bread, diced
1/2 tea. celery salt
1/2 tea. garlic salt
diced green pepper
1 tea. salt
1 cube margarine
chopped parsley

Mix everything together, and dump in oven casserole. Pour a cup of milk over the top, cover and bake one hour at 350.

I know, if you file that recipe away mentally under Pig Farm Potatoes, you'll probably never try them. So call 'em Ponderosa Potatoes. In fact, I bet Little Joe has a few pigs out behind the bunkhouse.

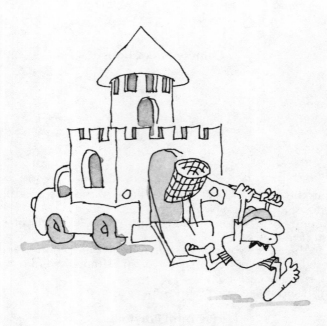

When Blaine Freer is afloat, the fish are in trouble. The Post-Intelligencer's resident Captain Ahab, Freer pursues our finned friends with a million-dollar camper, a thousand dollar boat and enough rods, reels and electronic depth-finders to single-handedly defeat the Russian trawler fleet.

Freer is also an amateur cook, brewer, winemarker, skier and bowler, so you can see he has a lot on his mind. When he is preoccupied with blackmouth, he is liable to absent-mindedly insert a herring dodger into the pencil sharpener. If the smelt are running at Kalaloch, he may emerge breathlessly from his camper with two (2) dipnets and no (0) pants.

When he is so preoccupied, conversations with him can be somewhat peculiar.

"Well, my wife has signed up for some Oriental cooking classes," he remarked recently, after fretting about a coffer dam on the Elwha.

"Is that right?" I responded cleverly. "Does she have a wok?"

"No," Freer said. "She'll drive the Volkswagen."

Which reminds me that I've got an easy recipe for Chinese noodles. Only it begins life as a British pork roast. Somewhere between supper on Sunday and dinner on Tuesday, east meets west.

English Pork Roast

Purchase a four-pound pork loin. Hopefully, the roast has been boned by your butcher. Because you are next supposed to put some thin onion slices into the pocket left by the bones. And if the bones are still there . . . well, I'd rather not be involved.

Rub the entire roast with a cut garlic clove, then coat with a mixture of salt, pepper and flour, the fat as well as the lean.

Chop up two onions, a carrot, some parsley and maybe a celery top, mix with 1/8 teaspoon of rosemary and 1/4 teaspoon of thyme. Glunk this mixture on the bottom of a pan, top with a rack, then the roast, fat side up. The vegetables should be lying there in a pile, directly under the roast, where they'll catch all the drippings.

Cook in a 350 oven for about an hour and 50 minutes, or until the thermometer announces that it is almost done.

Remove roast from oven, and turn heat to 400. Sprinkle the top part of the roast with two tablespoons brown sugar, return meat to oven for 15 minutes.

Remove roast to a hot platter. Pour off fat from pan and thicken remaining vegetables and drippings in the pan. What you thicken them with is two tablespoons of flour which have first been mixed until smooth with one tablespoon of soft butter. Add a cup of water, cook the gravy on top of the stove until thick, and serve with the roast and, oh, maybe some mashed potatoes and whatever.

That takes care of British Sunday. Now for the Chinese Tuesday.

Gung Ho Noodles for Four

Cook about eight ounces of Chinese egg noodles for 10 minutes in boiling salted water. Drain, then reheat the noodles in at least one quart of chicken broth or consomme, along with thin strips of the leftover pork, the more the merrier.

Serve in bowls, sprinkle with chopped green onions, pass the soy sauce and ring the dinner bell. Run, don't wok.

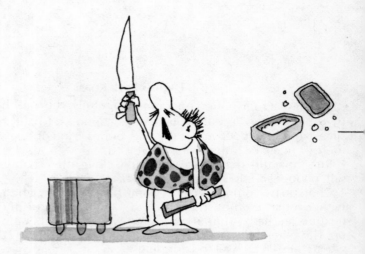

Know what is breaking up the American home?
Casseroles.

Don't give me a funny look, that statement is absolutely sound. I have suspected it was true for a number of years but lacked the necessary testimony to convert a premise into a promise.

And now that testimony is at hand, in the form of Lyall Watson's book, the Omnivorous Ape.

"Every week the senior hunter in every Western family commits ritual murder on the Sunday joint with a knife far larger than any carving knife needs to be," the author writes. "But it is more than just a carving knife, it is a stylized weapon that can only be wielded by the hunter."

It is the author's theory that modern man must fulfill some primeval drama that casts him as the hunter. He reaffirms his role with the carving knife, at the Sunday supper table. Woman was, originally, the scavenger of roots and berries. So today she gets to spoon up the creamed cauliflower. At least that is Watson's theory.

Aha, I ask, but what happens when she throws a casserole at her family, instead of a haunch of meat? The male is denied his dominant role.

Expect the mighty provider to pick out the bits of tuna fish with his carving knife? Who gets custody of the goulash, the hunter or the scavenger?

So long Renton, hello Reno. And all because of some macaroni.

And yet who can afford a respectable haunch of meat at today's prices? On second thought, you can't afford not to buy one, for the sake of your marriage.

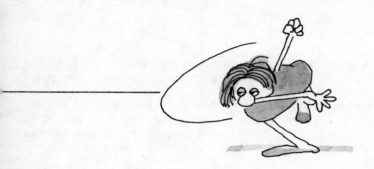

Primieval Leg of Lamb

Buy a leg of lamb. Preheat the oven to 350 degrees, while you are slicing up a half cup of carrots and a half cup of onions. Smash a couple of garlic cloves with an empty tokay bottle and add to the vegetables.

In another bowl mix together 1/4 teaspoon of ground rosemary, another clove mashed garlic, one tablespoon soy sauce, 1/2 cup dijon prepared mustard and four tablespoons vegetable oil. Use about one-third of this paste to completely cover the leg of lamb.

Remember the carrots and onions? OK, now plunk them into the center of your roasting pan and thunk the leg of lamb on top of them. If the vegetables are not completely covered by the lamb, they will quickly resemble some charred residue from the LaBrea tar pits.

Roast the lamb for 90 minutes, or until the meat thermometer reads 140 degrees. No, don't turn it or baste it or mess with it at all during the 90 minutes.

When the lamb is done, remove it to a hot platter and let it coast. Meanwhile, spoon most of the fat out of the roasting pan. Pour into the pan one and one-half cups of beef bouillon and boil for a few minutes, mashing and mushing the vegetables around a bit and scraping the bottom of the pan with a wooden spoon.

Remove the pan from the heat, and stir in the rest of that soy-mustard mess. Heat, strain into a sauce bowl and serve with the leg of lamb, which can be carved with either a three-foot machette or a blunt stone hatchet.

"Geez," a Phoenix hockey writer enthused, after the second period of a game in the Coliseum. "You guys have gone from last place to first place in the league, in one season."

And he wasn't talking about hockey. He had just finished a paper plate full of lasagne. And guess who was behind him in the press box chow line? It was Phil Maloney, then the coach of the Seattle team. He had delayed joining his players in the dressing room to mull over their so-far scoreless game.

"I saw the guy bringing this in before the game," Phil explained. Obviously, that's why he's a coach. If the players had been alert enough to notice something like that, they'd have been in the chow line, too, skates and all.

Sportswriters have their own rating system, for press box food. The Washington Huskies dropped one full grade the season they switched from cold chicken to pre-packaged hot dogs and sandwiches. How they manage to burn a hot dog bun black without disturbing the cellophane is another marvel of modern technology. Likely, the UW heats them in the school's nuclear whatzit.

The infrequent platter of lasagne definitely rates as big league eats, and other sports teams should acknowledge the benefits. As an example, after downing that big plate of lasagne, Phil Maloney went down on the ice and directed his team to three, third-period goals.

Now to be truthful, the average overstuffed sportswriter needs a half-time or second-period lunch about as much as he needs a 400-pound portable typewriter. In fact, they should post rules against feeding them, like in the rare bird house at the zoo.

Fortunately, The Post-Intelligencer's svelt hockey writer is often mistaken for a hockey stick except during the Longacres horse racing season, when people are constantly asking him who he's riding in the seventh race.

To keep his Irish heart humming we suggest the following between-periods snack, which also could be adopted for Fighting Irish football and Boston Celtic basketball.

Corned Big League and Cabbage

Rub a half cup of brown sugar into the hunk of corned beef, then place it in a pot with one and one-half cups water and a half-cup of dry white wine. Add to the pot:

1 chopped onion
1 tea. cloves
pinch dill
pinch of basil
pinch your wife
1 tea. dry mustard
8 peppercorns
pinch cinnamon
pinch caraway seed
1 tea. prepared horseradish

Bring everything to a boil, then cover and reduce heat. After you have simmered it for an hour, turn the meat, replace cover, and simmer for another 80 minutes.

Peel and halve some potatoes, turnips and carrots and toss into the pot. After 30 minutes add a head of cabbage, quartered, and cook just until the cabbage is tender, yet not wilted.

Serve the meat and vegetables on a big platter and pass remaining liquid from the pot around in a gravy bowl, to slosh over everything. Granted, because of all the spices this liquid looks kinda like old swamp water, but it tastes great.

In fact Phil Maloney might have two bowls, if the referee will kindly hold things up down there on the ice.

Occasionally you'll spot the item in a supermarket ad, under a heading like WAHOO, or HOWZABOUT THIS, or possibly PLENTY BIG DEAL.

HANGING TENDERS, $1.40 a pound.

"Hey, not bad!" you comment, under your breath. "But what in the name of Orville Faubus is a hanging tender?"

Had to ask, didn't you? That was your first mistake. Remember why you never buy sweetbreads? Because you looked up the definition.

According to the dictionary, a sweetbread is actually a calf thymus.

What's a calf thymus? Some lymphoid tissue.

Well, there went dinner.

Actually, you're going to have to engage in some culinary experimentation in these days of rising prices, because not everybody can afford to buy tenderloin (large internal muscle on each side of vertebrae column.)

And I can impart some information about the hanging tenders.

A butcher-shop informant, who talks out of the side of his mouth, rasped in a low voice: "There's just one in each beef."

Aha! The tail!

"Huh-uh," he corrected. "It hangs next to the kidney."

That's all you need to know. Pursue the subject and you're going to get hamburger tossed at you again for dinner.

The hanging tender looks like a perfectly respectable hunk of meat and can be prepared like so:

Hanging Tender

Mix together 1/4 cup soy sauce, 1/4 cup white wine, 1/4 cup oil, 1/2 teaspoon ginger, a minced clove of garlic and two tablespoons honey. Pour the marinade over the meat and let it sit for the better part of the day.

The hanging tender can either be grilled over a barbecue fire like a steak or broiled (about eight minutes to a side), in the oven, then sliced thinly.

The same marinade serves nicely for flank steak, too.

Everybody should have a hobby, but I'm not too sure about people who collect last year's lunch, in their refrigerator.

Know what's in that covered dish next to the eggs? Exactly two spoonfuls of pineapple yogurt. At least it was pineapple yogurt three months ago. You hesitate to throw it away because it's liable to come in handy, right? Handy for what? Rubbed on the tip of a pygmy arrow, it would probably stop a warthog dead in its tracks. But a myopic alleycat wouldn't touch it with a salad fork.

And what about those two boiled potatoes tossed on the bottom shelf after dinner last night?

Hmmm, we may need them after all, if that is actually a slab of leftover pot roast entangled in the aluminum foil. Oh, last week's corned beef, huh? It'll do:

Collector's Hash

Whack away at that hunk of cooked beef or corned beef until you have about three cups of diced cooked meat. And you'll want about two cupsful of diced cooked potatoes.

There should be a reasonably healthy onion hiding under that parsley. Chop up about 1-1/2 cups of onion and mince the parsley to get about three tablespoons.

Yeah, we'll need that green pepper. Slice it in half, throw away all the seeds and white pulp, chop the pepper and toss it into a big bowl, along with the meat, potatoes, onions and parsley.

Is that gravy or cinnamon sauce in the green bowl there? If it's gravy, pour it into the mixing bowl. If it's cinnamon sauce, shove it back into the refrigerator, and open a 10-ounce can of gravy.

Add one and a half teaspoons of salt, some freshly ground pepper, 1/4 teaspoon of thyme, one teaspoon of Worcestershire sauce. Mix everything into a big gloop.

Grease a two-quart casserole, fill with the hash and bake, covered, in a 375 oven for 45 minutes. Remove cover, cook another 15 minutes, and serve.

I think there's one stewed, leftover prune in that shot glass next to the tomato, if you demand dessert.

A guy doesn't have to sit down to a banquet every day, but he should be able to establish a simple standard of excellence in his abode. And this isn't a bad one to follow:

You should always eat better than your pet, unless it happens to be an argumentative gorilla.

This never used to be a problem. When the meal was over, you tossed a bone and a few leftover scraps to your dog, and if he didn't like it, he could always attempt to eat the cat.

In the modern supermarket of today, however, the pet food section occupies one solid wall and at first glance resembles Trader Vic's pantry.

It's possible to blow your beer money on Friskies Buffet or Kitty Stew. The catfood is called Mixed Grill, Gourmet Feast or a Mealtime for Finicky Appetites.

You can entice your cross-eyed mutt with dogfood called Chicken Stew or Roast Turkey or Lamb Chunks. You can stuff him full of Doggie Do Nuts or Dog Yummies or Home Style Stew. He can begin his day with Chicken, Liver and Bacon, and finish it with Meat N Egg Loaf.

And in between brunch and tea time, he'll dig up six tulips and wet on the rug.

Where does he get off demanding that people tickle his palate? What great contribution will the well-fed cat make to 20th century society? True, it may set a conference record for the slip-cover shred, but for that it deserves chopped sardines and canned salmon?

In an effort to keep one step ahead of your four-legged wastrel, you might whip up the following dish, which could be called Liver Flavored Feast, except that the catfood manufacturers have already copyrighted the name.

It has another advantage. Fry up a batch of aromatic liver and onions and you may well find yourself the object of Fluffy's full-fanged attack. Cooked in the oven, it is less liable to provoke an assault.

Baked People Liver

To serve three assemble:

6 slices liver
1/2 cup butter
1/4 cup chopped parsley
1 tea. salt
1/2 cup water
2 onions
1/2 cup red wine
1 tea. thyme
pepper
1/2 cup flour

Peel the onions, and whack into half-inch slices. Place in a baking dish, dot with butter. Assemble the wine, parsley, thyme, salt, pepper and 1/2 cup of water in a bowl and pour over the onion slices.

Cover the baking dish and bake in 350 oven for 30 minutes. Coat the liver with flour, place one hunk atop each large onion slice, replace cover and return to oven.

Cook for another 30 minutes, basting twice. Remove cover, cook 10 more minutes and then serve . . .

. . . After you have locked the cats in the basement.

Oven Spuds

Peel and slice three or four potatoes (again to serve three) in half lengthwise. Roll in two tablespoons olive oil and place face down in a pan. Sprinkle with a mixture of 3/4 teaspoon salt, some pepper, 1/2 teaspoon marjoram and a minced clove of garlic.

Pour any leftover olive oil over the spuds, fling the pan into the 350 oven for an hour and you're in business. The human-food business.

Homemade Jerky

Happen to have the right rear haunch of an elderly moose in your refrigerator meat drawer? If not, start searching for the cheapest LEAN slab of beef you can find, if you intend to make your own jerky.

Once I spotted some Argentine flank steak that was ridiculously cheap. Another time I found an inexpensive hunk of utility bottom round steak at Pike Place Market. Another market stall had a special price on an especially lean and boneless hunk of rump roast.

The point to be emphasized for jerky is that you do not need or want an expensive cut of meat. The low-graded U.S. Good and Utility will serve as well if not better. If you know of a horsemeat market or run across a special on old elephant tails, they would probably serve as well.

Trim as much fat from the meat as you can and then slice it into quarter-inch strips. I usually marinate the meat for a minimum of a day in:

1/4 cup soy sauce
1/4 tea. pepper
1/2 tea. onion powder
1/2 teaspoon liquid smoke
1 T. Worcestershire
1/4 tea. garlic powder
1 tea. season salt

When ready to cook, set oven at 175 degrees. Shake the excess moisture from the strips and string them out on cake racks or the oven racks, and let them cook slowly for five to six hours.

Remove from oven, blot the strips with a paper towel, cool, and then store in an old mayonnaise jar or plastic bags.

Cheapies–Sausages and Beans

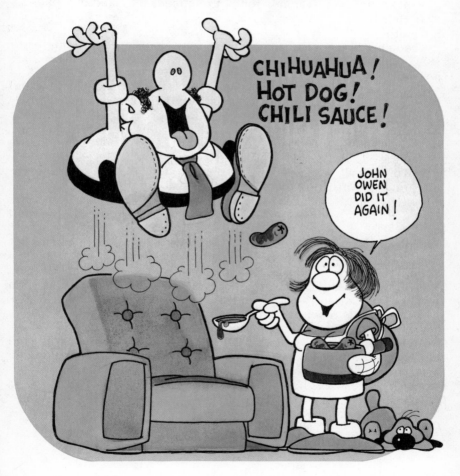

"Unlike any other 'canine,' the hot dog feeds the hand that bites it."
Heh. Heh.

Get it?

I certainly hope so. Chances are some advertising copywriter earns $87,000 a year and supports a mistress in Pawtucket, for dispensing such joviality for the NHDSC.

The NHDSC, as you might have guessed, is the National Hot Dog and Sausage Council, an insidious organization dedicated to the legal trafficking of the frankfurter. And, wow, are they doing a job. Between Memorial Day and Labor Day, Americans will consume 4-1/2 billion hot dogs, belch softly and groan, "I feel like I just et 4-1/2 billion hot dogs."

And the NHDSC isn't willing to rest there.

You may recall nothing significant about the fact that President Nixon's first trip to China took place in mid-February of 1972. Would you be stunned to learn that Feb. 17-26 was National Kraut and Frankfurter Week. And that kraut was discovered by the Chinese back in the third century B.C.?

Did you know that our new trade policy with Russia might involve hot dogs? The Soviet Union has requested technical advice from this country's leading producer of hot dogs. We send them Hot Dog Knowhow, they send us bauxite. Might not be a bad trade, after all. I often feel like I could stand a couple of teaspoons of bauxite and a warm glass of water, after two or three Coney Islands.

When I can locate a Coney Island.

An authentic Coney, known in some locales as the Chihuahua, is a red hot covered with chili sauce. But not just any chili sauce. It should bring a tear to your eye, warmth to your heart, produce a rumble in your stomach.

To manufacture a potful at home, follow these simple directions for:

Hooooooot! Dogs

8 onions
3 cloves garlic
3 tea. chili powder
3 cans mushroom spaghetti sauce
1 tea. salt
6 green peppers
1-1/2 lbs. hamburger
1 tea. cayenne

Peel and quarter the onions. Cut the peppers into quarters, discarding all the seeds and white pith. Peel the garlic cloves.

Now put the onions, peppers and garlic cloves through a food grinder. Sounds easy, right?

Wrong. I may be retarded, but my food grinder started to overflow with onion juice which began to form a lethal puddle on the kitchen floor and my eyes started watering and I couldn't blow my nose.

But I don't want to give away all my trade secrets.

When you have finally achieved a pile of onion-pepper pulp, you have the world by the ear on a downhill run.

Toss a quarter cube of margarine into a vat and when it melts dump in the onions and peppers and garlic. Cook, stirring, for about five minutes, over medium heat.

Add the ground beef, and smash everything up with a wooden spoon. Continue cooking, stirring, until the meat loses its redness.

Now fling in the canned spaghetti sauce and seasonings. Bring just to a boil, reduce heat and simmer 30 minutes. Taste and add more salt if you think it needs more salt.

This recipe makes approximately one ton of Coney Island sauce and you can store the surplus in the freezer.

What you do is put a hot dog (preferably grilled) in a warm bun. Heap with hot chili sauce, and enjoy.

Or, if you detest hot dogs, you can just pile a bunch of the Coney Island sauce into a bun for an eminently satisfactory Sloppy Joe.

But an official of the NHDSC will begin sticking frankfurter-shaped pins into a voodoo doll . . .

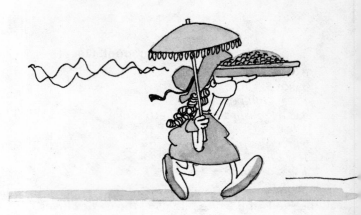

I could tell you how to spread one pound of sausage out over two meals, but that means you'd have to eat black-eyed peas for dinner, and I don't want to break up any families.

The black-eyed peas recipe was sent to me by a transplanted Southern housewife, who felt I had insulted the regional cuisine. She was probably mistaken. I happen to think black-eyed peas, dandelion greens, hominy grits and okra make for a fantastic feast, if you happen to be an Alabama cow.

It seems that the reason I've never fancied black-eyed peas is that I don't know how to prepare black-eyed peas, and the reader mailed in a prize-winning recipe from a magazine which had conducted a black-eye pea contest. It seems the way to properly cook black-eyed peas is to mess around with them until they no longer taste or look like black-eyed peas.

And I'll have to admit they're an improvement, served with . . .

But I'm ahead of myself. Half the sausage is reserved for Sunday's breakfast.

Sausage Cakes

The night before boil four potatoes until you can stick them with a fork without drawing blood. Sunday morning peel and chop the potatoes. Dump into a large bowl. Add the half-pound of bulk sausage, one-half of a small onion (grated), two slightly beaten eggs, 1/2 teaspoon salt, 1/8 teaspoon pepper and some chopped parsley for color.

Toss some dry bread into your blender to make one cup of fine crumbs. Spread them out on a piece of waxed paper.

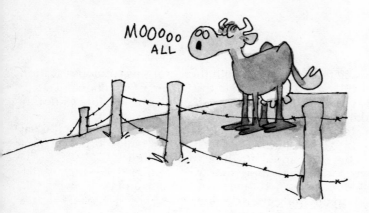

MOOooo ALL

Okay, now form the thoroughly mixed potato-sausage glunk into thick patties, and coat both sides in the bread crumbs.

Coat a skillet with hot oil and cook the patties over medium-low heat for 10 minutes, turn, cook another 10 to 15 minutes, and serve with tomato juice and buttered toast. It'll feed four.

Now use your imagination. Suppose you're having something dismal like ground beef patties or hot dogs or leftover heel-roast, for Sunday dinner. That's the time to hit your family with this authentic, Southern, grand prize vegetable side dish which, for some weird reason, the inventor calls:

Peasagne

Brown the remaining half-pound of sausage in a large saucepan and pour off the grease. Add one 15-ounce can of black-eyed peas, drained, a minced clove of garlic, a teaspoon of oregano and a teaspoon of basil.

Mash everything up in the pan. You can use your electric whirly-whazzit, a potato masher or a Don Mincher-autographed baseball bat.

When everything is smashed (except the cook) add a 15-ounce can of tomato paste, mix, and simmer, uncovered, for 30 minutes.

On second thought, never mind the wrinkled wieners, the ground beef patties or the second-hand roast. Those particular black-eyed peas would probably go great with some Southern Fried Chicken.

Especially since they no longer look or taste like black-eyed peas.

I don't know whether it still exists, but there was this fabulous vacation resort, see, which I think was located in the Bahamas. A millionaire ran it, and his idea was to let other people feel like millionaires, too. Curiously enough, he did it by eliminating money.

Oh, he didn't let the customers in free. What they did was to pay a flat fee, in advance. And then once they arrived at their fantastic, beach-front villa, they could have just about anything they desired.

See, they never had to think about money, once they'd paid their initial, and substantial, dues. They had their own barman, and their own cook, too. They could do anything they desired during the day, like sailing a yacht, fishing for marlin or diving for scubas. They could order anything for dinner, demand a vintage wine, and never see a check.

And a reporter for a magazine arrived at the resort to see how millionaires lived. He was either a terrific reporter, or else he was black-mailing the comptroller, to get such an assignment. But the magazine paid the full freight. The reporter and his wife were installed in their cottage, introduced to the hired help, and instructed to order anything they desired.

After three days, all they wanted to do was lie on the sand and eat tuna fish sandwiches.

They could go anywhere, do anything, feast like Renaissance kings. But once the novelty wore off, they just wanted to munch a tuna fish sandwich, and doze off to sleep in the sun.

That would happen to me, too. After three days I'd want a hot dog. Lord, I know what they're probably made from. I know all about the preservatives and the artificial coloring and the way the poor creatures are sometimes mistreated . . . drowned in warm water, then buried in a cold bun of a casket.

But grilled, spread with mustard, hot chili sauce and chopped onions, they are terrific, and after three days of oyster-stuffed steak under hollandaise sauce, I'd holler for a hot dog on my tropical isle. If pressed, I might even accept a bowl of:

Hot Dog Stew

1 onion
1 lb. hot dogs
1 cup tomato juice
1 T. Worcestershire
1 tea. chili powder
1/8 tea. garlic powder
large can kidney beans
1 green pepper
1 tea. salt
1 T. lemon juice
1 T. brown sugar
3 T. catsup
2 T. flour

Peel the onion and chop. Do the same to the green pepper, after removing pulp and seeds. Cut the dogs into bite-sized hunks. Heat a little oil in a large pot. Toss in the vegetables and dogs and cook over medium heat, stirring frequently.

When the wieners are beginning to look healthy and the vegetables are wilted, pour in all the liquids and seasonings, which have been thoroughly mixed with the flour. Cook over medium heat, stirring occasionally, until the sauce thickens, then add the beans, cover, reduce heat and let simmer about 20 minutes.

What's that? You say Hot Dog Stew doesn't sound like a tropical island delight? Then how about some:

Bean Soup Bahamas

Cut some hot dogs up into quarter-inch slices and saute lightly in some butter.

Meanwhile, open two cans of black bean soup. Mix in saucepan with two cups of milk, 1/8 teaspoon of Tabasco sauce and 1/2 teaspoon of ginger.

Using a mortar and pestel (made out of native stone) smash up two cloves of garlic and mix thoroughly with 1/2 cup of mayonnaise.

Stir this mixture into the soup, glunk in the hot dog slices and let the soup simmer (but not boil) for 20 minutes.

And see that the yacht is at my pier promptly at 10!

Sure, we all know that football pools are illegal, but you still might want to occasionally inquire about the point spread on Notre Dame-USC right? But you have to rely on information provided by others. Because you personally have no real measure of comparison.

That oversight has now been corrected. How? It's really simple. You've heard the nutritional axiom, "You are what you eat," right?

Well I happen to know what they eat! (Better make that two !!s.)

A couple of years ago I made a tour of PAC-8 football camps which included a training table lunch with the athletes. And I'll bet you never suspected before that the fleet Trojan halfback was one-half chicken, some chopped fruit and a dollop of mashed potatoes. Well he is, if my research is still valid. And that might tell you something about the Trojans. Before you make your bets, however, you should inspect the entire lineup.

WASHINGTON — Beef stroganoff on rice, cold ham, rolls, mixed salad and cake.

WASHINGTON ST. — Hot turkey sandwiches, mashed potatoes, green beans, assorted salads, soup and fruit.

USC — Fruit cocktail, one-half broiled chicken, mashed potatoes, green beans with almonds, rolls, ice cream.

UCLA — Luncheon steak, French fried onion rings, shrimp salad and strawberry pie.

CALIFORNIA — Clubhouse sandwiches and/or fish sticks, assorted salads and cherry tarts.

STANFORD — Hot beef sandwiches, mashed potatoes, green salad, apple pie alamode.

OREGON — French dip sandwiches, French fries, green beans, brownies.

OREGON ST. — Luncheon steak, French fries, salad, ice cream.

Well, there you have it. Now all you have to do is to try to figure out whether a French dip sandwich should rate a six-point edge over hot turkey. At first glance, it might appear that Oregon State and UCLA are destined for a 13-13 tie whenever they meet. But you're not going to overlook the onion rings, shrimp salad and strawberry pie, are you?

The emphasis on incidental details like these spell the difference between a good football team, and a great one. And a true football expert is one who knows how a cherry tart is going to measure up against a brownie, on third down and long yardage.

Personally, I don't play football, can't afford steak or shrimp, and my training table goes heavy on potatoes and knockwurst. Those are the main ingredients of the following dish, although smoked sausage or even top-quality hot dogs can replace the knockwurst, if you're forced to call an audible at the line of scrimmage.

Fourth Down
(Cause that's how many it'll serve)

1 can mushroom soup
1 small onion
1/4 cup green pepper
some pepper
1 lb. knockwurst
1/2 cup shredded cheese
1/2 cup milk
1/8 tea. savory
1/2 tea. salt
4 potatoes
margarine

Combine the cream of mushroom soup, the milk, chopped onion, green pepper, savory, salt and pepper.

Peel and thinly slice the potatoes. Cut the knockwurst into bite-sized pieces.

Grease a casserole. Line with half the sliced potatoes, top with half the knockwurst. Gloop half the soup mixture over the top. Add the rest of the potatoes, the rest of the knockwurst and the rest of the liquid. Dot with margarine, cover and bake in 350 oven for 75 minutes. Remove cover, sprinkle with cheese, and shove back into the oven, uncovered, for 15 minutes.

If you fumble the casserole halfway to the table, you might drive out to the University of Washington, and try to fake your way into line behind the coach. If you weigh 230 pounds and have a scab on the bridge of your nose, chances are he'll even help you to seconds.

147

The recipe for Beans Texian was entrusted to me by a gentleman named Guy Ham. Although he's a newspaper desk editor and a transplanted Texan, the only real thing I have against him is that whenever I encounter him in the hall I find myself saying, "Hi, Guy."

I suspect he gave me the recipe so that he'd have an excuse to set me straight on chili peppers. He maintains that their place in the diet of a country like Mexico is vital, and threefold. The peppers help preserve the meat, they supply some vitamins in a diet that is otherwise heavy on corn and beans. And, most important, the chilis create an appetite where none exists — like when it's 110 in the shade and a large dog has squatter's rights. Even on such a day the chili peppers beg — nay, demand — a diner's attention, Guy Ham proclaims.

Well, now I've got two things against him. Because he didn't mention the main reason most Mexicans, and some Texans, gleefully fling chili peppers into the pot.

It's so they can watch the gringos take a bite and go, "Aaaaahhhhgggg!"

The chili pepper is the principal form of entertainment, south of San Ygnacio, rivaling bullfights and mariachis. For some reason, the sight of a tourist with fried eyeballs, falling heavily to the restaurant floor, tongue protruding, is irresistible.

I offer as evidence the wrapper off a can of jalapeno peppers, which are featured in Guy Ham's Beans Texian. On one side of the can, it reads:

"Don Ramon suggests: A taste sensation for those who like extra hot peppers. Remove seeds from Old El Paso Hot Chili Peppers and soak in ice water for one hour. Drain and pat dry. Serve on relish tray."

Yeah, and then go let your tongue soak in ice water for an hour. Because jalapeno peppers are H-O-T although, as Ham points out, they taste like fire. That means they really don't change the flavor of the basic food which, in this case, consists of:

Hi Guy's Beans Texian

Trimming his original recipe to size and taste, I used one pound of small red beans and soaked them overnight. Guy Ham soaks them in a big green pot. I altered the recipe and used a big blue pot.

Proceeding as instructed, I added a little water so that the soaked beans were covered; then, five hours before dinner, turned on the fire and added three cut, but not minced, cloves of garlic, two chopped onions, two teaspoons of salt, one and a half teaspoons of both sage and thyme and one tablespoon of chili powder.

I added two canned jalapeno peppers, first removing seeds and chopping finely.

Bring everything to a boil, then turn heat to low and cover pot.

You can use almost any kind of meat with this dish, ham hocks, Spam or an old mule's tail, as little as a half pound or as much as a pound. I used about three-quarters of a pound of beef stewing chunks, first browning them on all sides in some hot oil in a skillet, then adding after the beans had cooked for about two hours.

If, after the full five hours of cooking time, the beans appear too soupy, bring them to a boil again until you've reduced the liquid, then serve. Guy Ham correctly suggests corn bread, avocado salad and beer, to go with the beans.

Chop up a few more of those canned jalapeno peppers and serve in a side dish. To experiment I added one chopped-up pepper to my second helping of beans and developed a brief case of the hiccups, which indicated the formula was near perfect.

It was hot, but I didn't have to soak my tongue in ice water for 60 minutes, as Don Ramon suggests.

Know how the hot dog was created? A concessionaire at the St. Louis Exposition of 1904 was in the habit of loaning white gloves to his customers, so that they could get a sanitary grip upon his steaming red hots. Apparently the customers were goaded into a life of crime by the temporary possession of one white glove. Because enough of them were stolen so the concessionaire had to seek another solution. Ergo, the bun!

First Aid for Franks

Add one tablespoon chopped onion, one-fourth teaspoon garlic salt, one-fourth teaspoon chili powder, two teaspoons of Worcestershire Sauce, two teaspoons molasses and one teaspoon prepared mustard to one cup tomato sauce.

Lightly brown split wieners in oil, then add the sauce and simmer 10 minutes. You can serve the wieners with mashed potatoes and white gloves. Or, you can dish them up with a generous helping of the sauce in warm, buttered buns.

Another RX for Dogs

Spread a package of wieners in the bottom of a casserole.

Open up a large can of a better-brand baked beans and toss them into another bowl. Add 1/4 cup molasses, one tablespoon prepared mustard, one tablespoon vinegar and a few drops of liquid smoke.

Pour this mess over the wieners in the casserole. Top with about six thin slides of onion and bake in a 350 oven until bubbling.

Did you know that Americans consume about 15 billion hot dogs a year. Stretched end to end, the wieners would reach the moon and back two and a half times. Sounds like a remarkable statistic until you sit back and reflect that 14.8 billion hot dogs probably produce more gas than a Saturn booster consumes in a month.

Foreign Dishes

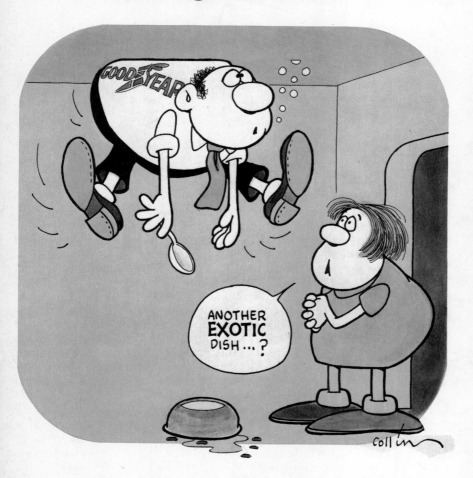

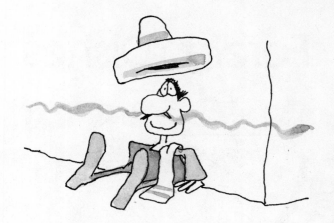

Mexico City was built too high, but is fortunately sinking, and nobody really minds because snails cost only 80 cents a pot.

This is just some of the incidental intelligence obtained by Your Correspondent at the XIX Olympiad in Mexico City.

Since the altitude of Mexico City is 7,350 feet, the broad jumpers soared like birds, and the distance runners fell down a lot.

The reason the city is slowly sinking is that it was thoughtfully built on a bog, which may be the reason the residents all walk softly and smile a lot.

They especially smile a lot around supper time, because the aroma is fantastic. The average American tourist arrives in Mexico City convinced his first meal will consist of a scrap of unwashed lettuce and a stomach pump. Not so. Mexico City has fantastic French, German, Swiss, Italian and Spanish restaurants. Also Mexican. Or you can order a pepperoni-and-cheese at Pizza Pete's, a haunch of rooster at the Kentucky Fried Colonel's or a stack of buckwheats at Aunt Jemima's.

But why should you, when snails are only 80 cents a pot, in that lazy little restaurant across from the British Embassy? They are covered with a Mexican sauce (the snails, not the British diplomats), you eat them with a tooth pick, and save a little space for the oysters piquant and crab bisque.

No, I am not going to suggest that you start Sunday morning off with a pot of snails. You're already starting to turn puce around the gills. And besides, your friendly neighborhood Soup-R-Save may be out of tooth-picks.

But for dinner you might consider some barbecued:

Carne Picarda de Vaca

All that means is "hamburger," but this particular dish sounds and tastes a whole lot better.

In advance, combine a pound of ground beef with a cup of minced onion, a cup of minced parsley, an egg, 1/4 cup of grated Parmesan cheese, 1/2 tablespoon salt and a sprinkling of pepper.

If you have a blender, toss in some dry bread, or else pulverize same with a rolling pin until you have a cup or more of fine crumbs. Spread them on some waxed paper.

Form the hamburger mixture into balls and flatten into cakes on the bread crumbs. Turn so the patties are coated with the crumbs on each side. They should be thin and about four inches in diameter.

Place on layers of waxed paper and chill in the refrigerator until you are ready to barbecue. It's best if you have a wide wire rack for your barbecue. Grease it, load up with patties and grill them over a medium fire about 2-3 minutes on each side. No longer.

Mexican Bean Pot

For the perfect side dish, construct the following:

Saute 1/2 cup minced onions in two tablespoons oil until soft. Combine onion in a pot with two cans of kidney beans, one cup canned tomatoes, a tablespoon of chili powder, a teaspoon of salt, a dash of liquid smoke.

Cook slowly on back of grill or stove. Dice 1-1/2 cups of cheddar cheese. When you have flipped the patties and are three minutes away from the dinner gong, toss the cheese into the bean pot and serve when melted. Feeds four.

See, you're smiling already!

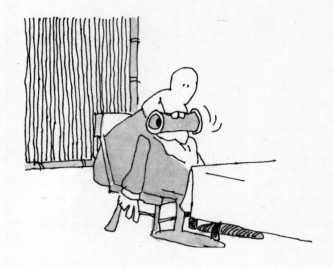

Don't get me wrong, I like Chinese food. I even like Chinese-German food although — according to the old saw — two hours later you're hungry again . . . for power.

My only complaint with Chinese food is that the average seven-course meal fails to build to a suitable climax. You begin the feast with shrimp-in-seaweed, advance through the 100-year eggs, the egg flower soup, baked fish in plum sauce, a heaping bowl of pork-mushroom-fried rice, mandarine duck lathered with orange sauce and, finally . . .

A fortune cookie.

Admit it, it's something of a comedown. When was the last time you turned to a fellow diner, slapped your forehead and exclaimed, "Wow, did you ever taste a better fortune cookie?"

Did anybody ever argue with you, "Hey, no, we don't wanna eat here. Let's walk six blocks to the Dragon's Breath. They've got these fantastic fortune cookies . . . "

Oh, I believe the message inside the cookies. But I'm pretty sure I could mistakenly munch the bamboo napkin holder, instead of the fortune cookie, on the way to the cash register and never be the wiser. Chinatown needs a better dessert, which is probably why fate brought me to this place, at this time.

But wait a minute. Before you get dessert, you've got to clean your supper plate, which happens to contain:

Onion-Pepper Beef

Buy a pound and a half of sirloin and cut it 1/2 inch thick (or if you know a market which carries sukiyaki beef, it's about the same thing). You'll also need:

4 cups sliced onions
1/2 tea. sugar
2 T. soy sauce
1 mashed clove garlic
1 green pepper
5 T. oil
2 T. sherry
2 T. cornstarch

Cut the green pepper in strips, discarding white pith and seeds. Heat half the oil in a skillet or wok and saute the onion and green pepper until they begin to soften. Add the sugar, one tablespoon soy sauce, one tablespoon sherry and the mashed garlic. Stir-cook 30 seconds and remove to heated plate.

Toss the beef strips with the remaining soy sauce, sherry and the two tablespoons of cornstarch. Pour rest of the oil into the skillet and when it is hot add the beef and stir-cook until browned.

Glunk the onion-pepper mixture back in the skillet, squoosh it around with the beef, let everything cook about two minutes and serve, maybe with some brown rice on the side.

Oh yeah, dessert. Well, I suppose we could call it:

Peking Parfait

Assemble four peaches grown either at Inner Mongolia or the Yakima Valley, whichever is closer. Peel and slice them.

Toss the peaches in a bowl with 1/2 cup of orange juice, three tablespoons of honey and two tablespoons of candied ginger, which has first been pulverized with a mortar and pestle. Let the bowl sit in the refrigerator for a couple of hours.

Then gloop a big spoonful of the peach mixture into the bottom of a parfait glass, add a couple of scoops of vanilla ice cream, with another big gloop of peach mixture on top. And if you really can't finish the meal without some sage oriental advice try this:

(Confucious say the Green Bay Packers may be susceptible to a quick kick on third down.)

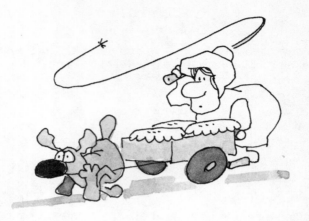

The sign appeared next to the till in a local cafeteria:

"HOMEMADE PIE NOW 45 CENTS DUE TO PRICE INCREASE AT THE BAKERY."

What bakery?

I had always assumed that the homemade pies were baked by a white-haired granny in Ballard and rushed downtown by dogcart after they had cooled briefly on the back stoop. I am reasonably certain that the Fair Trade Commission bestows an official frown on "homemade" pie which is the creation of a chrome computer-oven capable of spitting meringue to the far end of the conveyer belt.

Yet the practice is a common one.

Restaurant menus extoll the quality of homemade soup, homemade cake and home-fried chicken. Behind that chicken at a First Avenue beanery is an unshaven, gravy-splattered wretch exuding cigar ashes into the deep fat fryer. That steaming kitchen ain't "home" and he ain't "mother." Hopefully.

Chinese kitchens? They're something else, altogether. You never see the Hong Kong Cafe, the Four Seas or the Dynasty bragging about their "homemade Mandarin Duck" or urging some of "Grandma's Fortune Cookies" on you.

You see, to duplicate the output of even one small Chinese restaurant, your home had best come complete with a matched set of 15 concubines, each with her own chopping knife.

Obviously, it's cheaper — and a lot more peaceful — to eat in a restaurant. Either that, or discover some Chinese recipes which do not require six burners and eight cooks.

For example, you might prepare this side dish in advance:

156

Chinese Shrimp Salad

2 small cucumbers
2 T. salt
one small can shrimp
1 T. Oil
1/2 tea. sugar
1 T. soy sauce
1/2 tea. vinegar
1/4 tea. cayenne

Peel and shred the cucumbers. Sprinkle with the salt and let it sit there doing nothing for an hour or two. Rinse and drain.

Mix the cucumbers with the drained shrimp, the oil (olive or peanut), sugar, soy sauce, vinegar and cayenne. Let it cool off in the refrigerator while you construct the main course. Like the salad, it is also designed to serve four.

Homemade Almond Chicken

2 whole chicken breasts
3/4 tea. salt
2 T. cornstarch
3 T. soy sauce
1 tea. sugar
1/4 cup chicken bouillon
5 ounces sliced almonds
3 tea. peanut oil
one cup celery
one diced onion
1/2 cup bamboo shoots
1/2 cup water chestnuts
2 T. sherry

Skin and bone the chicken and cut into cubes. Mix the salt, cornstarch, soy and sugar and let the chicken cubes wallow around in this for 30 minutes.

Heat the oil in a skillet, toss in the chicken and saute until tender. Push the chicken to one side and saute the chopped celery, onion, bamboo shoots and water chestnuts, also until tender.

Add the chicken bouillon and sherry, moosh everything around in the pan with a wooden spoon as you reheat. Sprinkle with the sliced almonds and serve.

Maybe for dessert we could have some homemade ice cream from Tradewell.

For some reason, the host of reporters and commentators who accompanied Richard Nixon on his historic first trip to China failed to grasp the significance of the journey and ignored the enormous coup scored by our diplomatic corps.

We were finally able to unload those weird musk oxen.

Maybe it escaped your notice, too. We shipped two San Francisco musk oxen as a gift to the people of China, receiving in return a matched set of giant pandas.

I never did get a good look at the pandas, but one of the television networks showed some film footage on the oxen. I wouldn't want to accuse the government of passing off factory seconds on the Chinese people. But this one ox kept running head first into a tree, and appeared the intellectual inferior of the average rubber eraser.

I believe former vice president Agnew had unsuccessfully offered it to the National Press Club as a mascot and later smuggled it aboard a hijacked jet to Cuba, only to have it returned by Castro, C.O.D.

So State Department dealt it to China on a fast shuffle, and sent along a mate. After three generations there shouldn't be a tree left in China.

Maybe it's a fair swap. Over the years the Chinese have sent to this country chop suey, egg foo yung, chow mein and a lot of other dishes they wouldn't touch with a 10-foot chop stick.

One of the television commentators on Nixon's First Trip reported that he encountered all sorts of exotic Oriental food, but nothing that he had ever spotted on the menu of a Chinese restaurant in this country.

Don't know whether Mongolian Hot Pot is included in this blanket indictment. I'd always assumed it originated in the general vicinity of Mongolia, but I'll probably learn it was born at an Italian restaurant in Austin, Texas, the day they ran out of raviolis.

In any event, it provides another use for that fondue pot you never got around to trying. And it's an interesting company dish, only moderately expensive and surprisingly easy to prepare, provided you have 700 million Chinese in your kitchen that day to chop the ingredients into bite-sized pieces.

Mongolian Hot Pot

Say you're going to have about eight guests. Buy a large flank steak, slice it in half with the grain, then carve against the grain into a stack of quarter-inch slices of raw beef.

Skin and bone four chicken breasts, and carve them into quarter-inch slices. Some raw prawns, shelled, cleaned and sliced in half lengthwise, might go good, too. Whack some fresh mushrooms into quarters, assemble some raw spinach leaves, hunks of Chinese cabbage, maybe some snow peas or leaf lettuce.

Heat some chicken bouillon in a large pot and when it boils, ladle into the fondue pot or pots. Four diners for one pot is about right, but a chafing dish will accommodate more, if you have one.

Arm each guest with a few bamboo skewers, pass the plates of food, and let everyone help himself to a variety.

They're on their own from this point, threading the food on skewers, cooking in the bubbling bouillon for a minute or so, then dipping into a variety of sauces . . . maybe some hot Chinese mustard, the plum sauce available in Chinese markets, a teriyaki sauce which is half soy, half sherry with a sprinkling of garlic salt and ginger. Add hot bouillon from the big pot as needed.

When the meat, chicken and prawns are about exhausted, toss the remaining vegetables into the pots of bouillon, along with some thin Chinese noodles and maybe a bit of soy sauce. Cook until the noodles are soft and then serve in soup plates as a final course.

Oh, sure, you can serve some green tea if you wish, but we'll probably learn next week that the root beer float is the Chinese national drink.

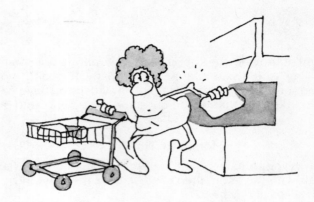

It's a wonder that science has never conducted research into a specific and remarkable phenomenon of nature. In fact, I have never actually seen the subject discussed in print, although virtually every consumer knows that the premise is absolutely sound.

To wit: It is absolutely impossible for the human hand to transfer a package of choice veal cuts from the meat market cooler into a plain, metal shopping cart.

Oh, you can get it halfway there. And then your elbow involuntarily locks. Absolutely nothing you can do about it. It's an unexplainable quirk of physiology.

Well, there may be a partial explanation, in the hieroglyphics inscribed on the right-hand edge of the label, where it reads:

VEAL SCALLOPS $3.67 lb.

You're into your butcher about $5 for some raggedy cuts of meat which can be transformed into an acceptable veal scallopini only with considerable aid from tomato sauce and Parmesan cheese. Is it possible that the roots of the Mafia can be traced to $3.67 veal? Was Al Capone motivated by nothing more than a gnawing hunger for a little veal marsala?

It's possible, because we recently tested the locked-elbow theory again at a Seattle supermarket. The veal was snatched from the case and thrust rapidly toward the shopping basket.

But guess what landed in the bottom? A $1.61 packet of boneless pork cutlets. So long, Italy. Hello, Hong Kong.

Sweet and Sour Pork

Trim the fat from pork cutlets to serve four and cut into three-quarter inch cubes. Then you'll need: 2 eggs, 4 tablespoons sugar, 2 tablespoons sherry, 1/2 teaspoon salt, 4 tablespoons oil, seasoned flour, 2 cloves garlic, 1 cup pineapple juice, 4 tablespoons vinegar, 2 tablespoons cornstarch and 2 tablespoons soy sauce.

Split the garlic cloves, saute in hot oil, then remove when they darken.

Dip the cubed pork into seasoned flour and then in beaten eggs. Fry in hot oil until golden brown, then drain and plop into a warmed dish or platter in a slow oven.

Mix cornstarch and sherry in a saucepan. Toss in the sugar, salt, sherry, juice, vinegar and soy sauce and boil until thickened. Pour over the pork and serve.

However, if you encounter another portion of the Chinese pig consider:

Pork Slices

Purchase a pork tenderloin, if you can find one, otherwise use lean pork shoulder. If you use the tenderloin, about a pound and a quarter in size, cut it in half lengthwise so you have two long pieces of meat, about an inch square. Marinate for at least four hours in the following mixture:

   1/2 cup soy sauce
   1/4 tea. salt
   1/2 tea. garlic powder
   1/2 cup sugar

At meal time, broil the drained meat six inches from heat for about 25 minutes, turning about every five minutes. If the outside begins to char during the later stages of cooking, lower the oven heat to about 450 for the remainder of the 25-minute cooking time.

Slice the pork diagonally into bite-sized pieces, which can be dipped in oven-toasted sesame seeds, some hot Chinese mustard or a soy-white wine mixture.

What's with this luau jazz?

Suddenly, everybody seems to have come down with a bad case of island fever. Everywhere you turn, somebody is throwing a luau. You can hear native drums beating softly outside the Eagles Club. Electric guitars twang softly at PTA potlucks. The Moose Lodge banquet room is transformed into a plastic paradise for a Totems Booster Club hockey bash.

Maybe we'd better make only passing mention of the Totem Boosters Authentic South Seas Luau a couple of years ago, since it went off as smoothly as the landing on Guadalcanal. Depending upon which officer of the club you listened to, the guests did or did not eat the decorations, they did or did not insult the hula dancers and the entertainment chairman did or did not stick pins into a voodoo doll of a Totem forward.

The turmoil was predictable. Genuine Northwest Totems relate to Allakaket or Shaktoolik, rather than Ponape.

If the Totem Boosters want to throw an authentic bash, they should slice up some seal blubber.

What's the big deal about poi? Let some Cream of Wheat go bad on you, and you've got the same thing.

Of course, if somebody is roasting a suckling pig over a banana frond fire while wahines undulate wantonly in the background, you might give me a call. But I suspect they make-do with some fried rice, ginger beer and a scratchy Don Ho record of Wakanakalaka Meter Maid, at your average Seattle luau.

If you really want to sample a South Seas staple, you might stay home and cook up a pot of this authentic native dish which is prepared with two pounds of Kansas City beef and a packet of gravy mix packaged by some Poles in East Orange, New York.

Luau-wow!

2 lbs. bottom round
2 T. cooking oil
1 packet gravy mix
1/2 cup red wine
flour
1 onion
1 can beef bouillon
6 oz. pineapple juice

Cut meat into serving-sized pieces. Sprinkle with flour and pound with the dull side of your butcher knife, or an authentic South Seas machete.

Brown meat on both sides in oil, which has been preheated in a Dutch oven. Add sliced onion and stir-cook until it is soft. Mix gravy powder with the bouillon, wine and pineapple juice, and pour over the meat.

Bake uncovered for two and a half hours in a 325 oven.

You might serve with rice and:

Oriental Broccoli

Wash two pounds of broccoli and cut off the tough ends. Cut stalks into diagonal half-inch slices.

Heat three tablespoons cooking oil in skillet, add two minced cloves garlic, cook briefly but don't brown, dump in the broccoli and sprinkle with 1/2 teaspoon ground ginger and one teaspoon salt. Stir-cook two minutes, add a cup of chicken bouillon, cover and cook two more minutes.

While this is happening, mix four teaspoons cornstarch with four teaspoons water and four teaspoons soy sauce.

Remove cover from skillet and stir in the cornstarch-soy mixture until it thickens.

And if you really need native drums with dinner, turn on the revolving clothes drier, and toss in a couple of sneakers.

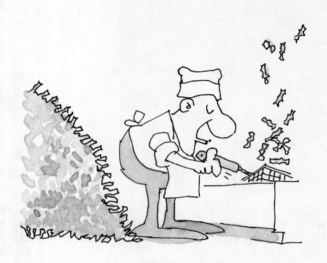

Rumor has it that Sir Walter Raleigh discovered the potato in the West Indies, and eventually introduced it to the British Isles.

But a terrible thing happened to the potato, before it was returned to the Americas. Some nert boiled it in oil.

And it is quite possible that today, the resultant French fry poses a greater threat to these United States than pollution, revolution or the nuclear bomb.

From Tuscarora, Me., to Twisp, Wash., a veritable army of wretched fry cooks are this moment heating up the oil and rattling their baskets in anticipation. They'll shortly be serving up a mountain of French fries that are half-cooked, spaghetti limp, oozing with grease and completely indigestible. They'll dish them up with hot dogs, fried fish, burgers rare and pronto pups.

At this moment a million stomachs are rumbling in futile protest.

The curse is not limited to America. The British bolt them down, but look at the state England is in. I am forced to report than they even consume French fries in France.

But there are still outposts of resistance. Like the humble Scottish cottages where somebody's mum is whipping up some champ.

"Champ" is Scottish for "mash" or "grind" and during the lean years mash potatoes were often the appetizer, the entree and the dessert.

Scottish Champ

Boil six peeled potatoes in salted water. In another pan plunk two cups of milk, four tablespoons of butter and about 20 green onions, cut into tiny pieces. Simmer until soft.

Drain the potatoes and mash, using the milk-onion mixture for the moisture, and adding salt to taste. You are required by law to create a canyon in the champ when it is dished up on your plate, filling the void with a man-made reservoir of butter.

Or, if your bus leaves in 10 minutes, you can simmer some cut-up green onions in the water-milk-butter-salt mixture specified on your instant potato box, whirl the mixture briefly in a blender and proceed as instructed.

Since times aren't THAT tough, you can serve this up with, ohh, maybe some cold meat loaf. Which means you are probably going to have to first construct some hot meat loaf.

Spicy Meat Loaf

Mix 1-1/2 pounds of hamburger with a cup of parmesan cheese, 1/2 cup chopped green pepper, 1/2 cup chopped onion, a cup of cracker crumbs, one egg slightly beaten, 3/4 cup milk and 1 teaspoon of salt.

Bake in a bread pan 45 minutes at 350. Plop the loaf out onto a baking sheet and coat all sides with a mixture of 3/4 cup catsup, 1/4 teaspoon Tabasco, 1 tablespoon chili powder and 1/2 tablespoon oregano. Bake another 15 minutes and serve.

But not with French fries.

It seems to me the Irish get an awful lot of distance out of corned beef and cabbage, considering that it is a pretty poor substitute for lasagne.

Yet each year the Irish-Americans get their funny bow ties out of their dresser drawers, they put on a pair of green socks, and more or less demand that everybody smell up their kitchen with a pot of corned beef and cabbage.

How about equal time for the Italian-Americans? For some reason their native land consists of one big tantalizing aroma. They are responsible for spaghetti, pepperoni pizza, fettuccine, Mozzarella and prosciutto, yet they hardly ever get to strut their stuff. Corned beef and cabbage, indeed!

Not only that, but most Americans are ashamed to be caught with a dollop of spaghetti sauce on their lip, because there is some myth about pasta being fattening. It's actually an excellent diet food. (You say you've seen some overweight Italians? Whew! You should see the size they get if they quit eating pasta!)

What the Italian-Americans really need is a holiday, and don't throw Columbus Day at me. What did you have to eat last Columbus Day? See, a complete blank.

I have seized upon two possible dates for the new national holiday.

May 15, 1796 was the day Napoleon's army marched in Milan, and Lord knows he must have worked up a hunger. But May 15 is pretty close to Easter and I think maybe we'd better spread our holidays out a little better than that.

So I have settled on June 2. Fortunately, June 2, 1800, was the date Napoleon occupied Milan for a second time.

The standard menu for Napoleon Day should begin with antipasto, minestrone, work through the spaghetti, a few meatballs and conclude with Italian fried chicken and an enormous slab of:

Napoleon Day Lasagne

4 slices bacon
1 chopped onion
1 chopped carrot
1 chopped rib celery
3/4 lb. ground beef
1 cup beef stock
1-1/2 cups cottage cheese
1/2 cup dry white wine
1/2 cup tomato paste
salt, pepper
1/2 tea. Italian seasonings
10 broad lasagne noodles
1/2 lb. Mozzarella
1/4 cup grated Parmesan

Dice bacon and saute in two tablespoons butter until lightly browned. Add the chopped onion, carrot and celery. Cook until vegetables begin to soften, then toss in the ground beef.

Brown the meat, breaking it up with a fork. Add the beef stock, wine, tomato paste, salt, pepper and Italian seasonings. Cover and simmer 40 minutes.

Cook the 10 broad lasagne noodles in boiling salted water until tender, about 25 minutes.

Layer half the meat sauce in the bottom of a big oven dish. Top with five pieces lasagne, half the Mozzarella cheese, thinly sliced, and dot with 3/4 cup cottage cheese. Then add a second layer of meat sauce, noodles, Mozzarella, cottage cheese and finally top with the grated Parmesan.

Cook 30 to 40 minutes in a 350 oven.

Hmm, that sounds pretty good. Let's see, tradition also dictates that the meal should be accompanied by a bottle of Chianti and concluded with a snifter of Napoleon brandy.

And put the leftovers in a doggie bag, if you have any needy Irish friends.

Johnny O'Brien claims he comes from a community so small the head of the Mafia is a Filipino.

I'm glad he said it, instead of me. Because I have a lurking suspicion I am still high on the enemies' list of the Daughters of Italy.

Merely intending to pass along the particulars of an Italian dinner in my newspaper column, I made the mistake of suggesting that it be served with a bottle of Da . . .

Oops, almost did it again. What I should have suggested was a bottle of "homemade Chianti." The term I used prompted a flurry of angry phone calls from offended Italian women.

"Gee, I'm sorry," I usually responded. "no offense was intended. I've heard the term used so freely — sometimes by friends of Italian parentage — that I honestly didn't think it was objectionable."

"You must associate with a low class of Italians . . . " one lady fumed.

"Well, I have associated with Edo Vanni, but he always assured me he was a high-class Italian. Speaking of "homemade Chianti," Edo once confided that wine was served with meals daily at his home. "I couldn't wait until I turned 21, so I could quit drinking," Edo swore.

Restauranteer Bill Gasperetti likes me well enough to confide the source of his Italian sausage. John Boitano hasn't thrown me out of any of his football games, yet. Heck, I once even attended a Daughters of Italy banquet.

"Why don't you come up with some recipes for zucchini?" recently asked another high-class Italian friend, Lou Guzzo.

Then five minutes later, he advised, "One thing you should never do is try to tell an Italian how to cook zucchini . . . "

Sheeee! That's those Italians for you.

For what it's worth, here's how they should cook zucchini.

Sunrise in Naples

To serve brunch to three, select one medium-sized zucchini, trim off the ends and slice, without peeling. Cook in boiling salted water for two minutes, and immediately drain.

Peel and chop one small onion, and saute until soft. Chop up three cherry tomatoes.

Layer the bottom of an oven casserole with the zucchini, sprinkle with salt and pepper and dab with butter. Dump the onion and tomato bits on top.

Beat four eggs with 1/4 cup milk, salt, pepper and a sprinkling of cayenne pepper.

Pour the eggs over the zucchini-onion mixture, sprinkle generously with grated parmesan cheese and bake in a 450 oven for 15 minutes.

Six hours later you'll be ready for a main dish, again to serve three, which you can call:

Sunset in Sicily

6 strips bacon
1 large zucchini
salt, pepper
2 cups cooked meat
2 cups chicken broth
1/2 cup Monterey Jack cheese
1 large onion
olive oil
1/4 cup milk
2 T. butter
3 T. flour

You can use any leftover meat for this dish. Mrs. Eater, who prepared it, used lamb, but beef or ham would serve just as well.

Cut bacon in strips and fry almost, but not quite, to the point of crispness. Remove bacon, and saute the chopped onion in the bacon fat, until soft.

Chop ends off the zucchini, slice (without peeling) and saute lightly on both sides in another skillet, coated with olive oil.

Put one tablespoon olive oil in bottom of an oven casserole. Top with layer of zucchini slices, salt, pepper, some meat, some onions, then more zucchini, meat, onions, so forth until you come to the final layer, which must be zucchini.

In a saucepan briefly stir-cook two tablespoons butter with three tablespoons flour. Pour in two cups boiling chicken broth. Stir-cook until it thickens, remove from heat, add 1/4 cup milk and slop everything into casserole. Top with the grated jack cheese and toss into 350 oven 30 minutes.

And serve with a cold bottle of Dr. Pepper.

Two-Day Spaghetti and Meatballs

No, it doesn't take you two days to eat them, but almost. The name refers to the fact that you can split the cooking process into two parts, if that is going to make life simpler for you.

Like on Wednesday you can construct the sauce, collecting:

1 minced onion
1 minced stalk celery
large can tomatoes
large can tomato sauce
1/2 cup red wine
1 cup water
3 T. minced green pepper
1 minced clove garlic
3 T. oil
1 tea. oregano
1 T. basil
2 tea. salt

Saute the vegetables and garlic in oil until wilted. Add tomatoes, the tomato sauce, oregano and basil, simmer one hour, stirring occasionally. Add wine, water, salt and a good grinding of pepper and cook another hour.

Then like on Thursday you can assemble:

2 lbs. ground beef
1 minced clove garlic
1/3 cup parmesan
1 cup dry bread crumbs
1/4 cup chopped parsley
1/2 cup olive oil
1 chopped onion
4 eggs
1/8 tea. oregano
1 tea. salt
1/2 tea. pepper

Mix the meat with the onions, garlic, cheese, crumbs, eggs, parsley, oregano, salt and pepper. Form into medium meatballs. Brown in hot oil, draining on paper towels as each batch is cooked.

Reheat the spaghetti sauce, dump in the meatballs and when everything is steaming hot serve with about a pound and a half of cooked spaghetti, to amply serve six.

There may even be a meatball left over for the cat.

INDEX

Meatball Stew 95
Sasquatch Steak 91
Spicy Meat Loaf 165
Sweet Pea's Meatballs 95
Gung Ho Pork Noodles 129
Ham and Egg Pie 9
Hamburgers 19
Hanging Tender 134
Henry VIII Pot Roast 117
Hi Guy's Beans Texian 149
Hood Canal Stew 45
Hooooot Dogs 141
Hot Dog
Another RX for Dogs 150
First Aid for Franks 150
Fourth Down 147
Stew 145
Hot Pot 119
Hungarian Goulash 99
Italian Sunrise 10
Kidneys, Curried 6
Lamb, Leg 131
Lasagne 167
Liver, Baked 137
Luau-wow 163
Marinades 108, 109
Market Mallard 87
Massage Parlor Stew 121
Meat Loaf 165
Meatballs
Gingered 15
Soup 35
Stew 95
Sweet Pea's 95
Mexican Bean Pot 153
Mexican Pot Roast 113
Mongolian Hot Pot 159
Mushrooms
Cocktail 93
Sherried 15
Napoleon Day Lasagne 167
Omelet
Old China 7
Zucchini 8
Onion-Pepper Beef 155
Onion Soup 27
Oven Spuds 137
Oysters
Mafia 47
Sherried 47
Stew 49
Peasagne 143
Peking Parfait 155
Pheasant 88
Pig Farm Potatoes 127
Pike Place Soup 31
Pizza 17

Pork
Chinese Chops 127
Chops 127
English Roast 129
Noodles 129
Peasagne 143
Sausage Cakes 142
Sandwiches 20
Slices 161
Sweet and Sour 161
With Clams 41
Potatoes
Balls 65
Caraway Salad 125
Champ 165
Cheesed 82
Curry-Fried 10
Grated 64
New 63
Oven Spuds 137
Pan Cakes 57
Pig Farm 127
Pot of Roast 115
Primieval Leg of Lamb 131
Puget Sound Gutbuster 43
Ranchhouse Roundsteak 101
Rice
Giblet 88
Parmesan 90
With Peas 105
Salad
Caraway Potato 125
Garlic Crouton 107
Salmon
Apple Jack 59
Seattle BBQ 59
Sandwich, Breakfast 11
Sasquatch Steak 91
Sausage Cakes 142
Scipio's Soup 36
Scottish Champ 165
Seagoing Spaghetti 55
Senta-Cheese Berger 22
Sherry-Soy Steak 111
Sherried Mushrooms 15
Shrimp Chowder 36
Shrimp Salad Chinese 157
Shrimp Soup 29
So Long Soup 25
Son-a-Gun Stew 123
SOS Rarebit 7
Spaghetti and Meatballs 170
Spaghetti, Seagoing 55
Spareribs 125
Spicy Meat Loaf 165
Split Pea Soup 25
Steak Soup 35

GOURMET GIZZARDS

1 med. diced onion
1 large stalk celery, diced
1 lb chick gizzards
1 lb chicken backs & necks
Salt, pepper, paprika & MSG
1 lb hamburger
1 minced garlic clove
1/4 c beef bouillon

Toss onions and celery in skillet covered with hot oil and when vegetables begin to soften, remove from pan. Brown giblets and chicken pieces in the same pan, in 2 batches, sprinkling with salt, pepper, paprika & MSG.
Meanwhile mix hamburger with garlic, 1 t salt, some pepper, the beef stock and 1/4 t MSG. Mix thoroughly & then form hamburger into small meatballs.
Dump giblets and vegetables into an oven pot or casserole. Pour the sauce over the top, then toss in the meatballs, cover and cook for 3 hrs at 275° oven. You can fish out the more prominent chicken bones before serving if you want or let cool, remove bones & reheat. It improves overnight.

<u>CREAMY SAUCE</u> (which isn't, really)

1 undiluted can tomato soup
1 bottle chili sauce

½ c water
1 T vinegar
¼ c lemon juice
1 T Worcestershire
⅓ c brown sugar
1 t seal. pepper , ¼ t MSG

Mix all together before pouring over
giblets. Makes a great dinner served
with noodles and salad.

Printed by University Printing Company